Department of Veterans Affairs
Health Services Research & Development Service | Evidence-based Synthesis Program

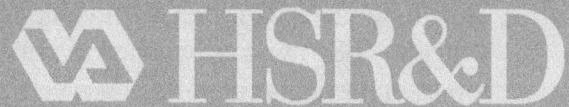 

Efficacy of Complementary and Alternative Medicine Therapies for Posttraumatic Stress Disorder

I0470878

August 2011

Prepared for:

Department of Veterans Affairs
Veterans Health Administration
Health Services Research & Development Service
Washington, DC 20420

Prepared by:

Evidence-based Synthesis Program (ESP) Center
Durham Veterans Affairs Healthcare System
Durham, NC
John W Williams Jr., M.D., M.H.Sc, Director

Investigators:

Principal Investigator:
Jennifer L. Strauss, Ph.D.

Co-Investigators:
Remy Coeytaux, M.D., Ph.D.
Jennifer McDuffie, Ph.D.
John W. Williams Jr., M.D., M.H.Sc

Research Associate:
Avishek Nagi, M.S.

Medical Editor:
Liz Wing, M.A.

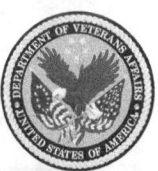

PREFACE

Health Services Research & Development Service's (HSR&D's) Evidence-based Synthesis Program (ESP) was established to provide timely and accurate syntheses of targeted healthcare topics of particular importance to Veterans Affairs (VA) managers and policymakers, as they work to improve the health and healthcare of Veterans. The ESP disseminates these reports throughout VA.

HSR&D provides funding for four ESP Centers and each Center has an active VA affiliation. The ESP Centers generate evidence syntheses on important clinical practice topics, and these reports help:

- develop clinical policies informed by evidence,

- guide the implementation of effective services to improve patient outcomes and to support VA clinical practice guidelines and performance measures, and

- set the direction for future research to address gaps in clinical knowledge.

In 2009, the ESP Coordinating Center was created to expand the capacity of HSR&D Central Office and the four ESP sites by developing and maintaining program processes. In addition, the Center established a Steering Committee comprised of HSR&D field-based investigators, VA Patient Care Services, Office of Quality and Performance, and Veterans Integrated Service Networks (VISN) Clinical Management Officers. The Steering Committee provides program oversight, guides strategic planning, coordinates dissemination activities, and develops collaborations with VA leadership to identify new ESP topics of importance to Veterans and the VA healthcare system.

Comments on this evidence report are welcome and can be sent to Nicole Floyd, ESP Coordinating Center Program Manager, at nicole.floyd@va.gov.

Recommended citation: Strauss JL, Coeytaux R, McDuffie J, Nagi A, Williams JW Jr. Efficacy of Complementary and Alternative Therapies for Posttraumatic Stress Disorder. VA-ESP Project #09-010; 2011.

This report is based on research conducted by the Evidence-based Synthesis Program (ESP) Center located at the Durham VA Medical Center, Durham, NC, funded by the Department of Veterans Affairs, Veterans Health Administration, Office of Research and Development, Health Services Research and Development. The findings and conclusions in this document are those of the author(s) who are responsible for its contents; the findings and conclusions do not necessarily represent the views of the Department of Veterans Affairs or the United States government. Therefore, no statement in this article should be construed as an official position of the Department of Veterans Affairs. No investigators have any affiliations or financial involvement (e.g., employment, consultancies, honoraria, stock ownership or options, expert testimony, grants or patents received or pending, or royalties) that conflict with material presented in the report.

TABLE OF CONTENTS

FIGURES

TABLES

EXECUTIVE SUMMARY

BACKGROUND

Posttraumatic stress disorder (PTSD) is the emotional disorder most frequently associated with combat and other potentially traumatic experiences that may occur during military service. It is often chronic and may be associated with significant comorbidities and functional impairments. Current first-line PTSD therapies include trauma-focused cognitive behavioral psychotherapies, stress inoculation training, and pharmacotherapies. Complementary and alternative medicine (CAM) interventions include a range of therapies that are not considered standard to the practice of medicine in the U.S. CAM therapies are widely used by mental health consumers, including Veterans, and numerous stakeholders have expressed strong interest in fostering the evidence base for these approaches in PTSD. Thus, this evidence synthesis was requested by VA Research and Development to inform decisions on the need for research in this area. Four key questions (KQs) guided this systematic review:

KQ 1. In adults with PTSD, are mind-body complementary and alternative medicine therapies (e.g., acupuncture, yoga, meditation) more efficacious than control for PTSD symptoms and health-related quality of life?

KQ 2. In adults with PTSD, are manipulative and body-based complementary and alternative medicine therapies (e.g., spinal manipulation, massage) more efficacious than control for PTSD symptoms and health-related quality of life?

KQ 3. In adults with PTSD, are complementary and alternative medicine therapies that are movement-based or involve energy therapies more efficacious than control for PTSD symptoms and health-related quality of life?

KQ 4. For treatments evaluated in KQs 1–3 that lack randomized controlled trials, is there evidence from other study designs that suggests the potential for treatment efficacy?

METHODS

We searched peer-reviewed, English-language publications in MEDLINE® (via PubMed®), Embase®, PsycINFO®, Cumulative Index to Nursing and Allied Health Literature® (CINAHL), and the Cochrane Controlled Trials Registry from database inception through December 22, 2010. Standard search terms, developed in consultation with a master librarian, targeted CAM therapies (e.g., acupuncture, mind-body, meditation), PTSD, and randomized controlled trials (RCTs) in adults. We searched the Published International Literature on Traumatic Stress (PILOTS) database (April 26, 2011), a specialized PTSD database maintained by the National Center for Posttraumatic Stress Disorder, to identify existing systematic reviews and studies of relaxation treatments and identified additional studies from reference lists of included studies and review articles. We included RCTs comparing an eligible CAM treatment to control or standard treatment for adults with PTSD. When RCTs were not identified, we searched for relevant prospective studies. Titles, abstracts, and articles were reviewed in duplicate, and relevant data were abstracted by the authors, all of whom have been trained in the critical analysis of empirical literature. To identify relevant studies in progress, or completed but unpublished studies, we searched ClinicalTrials.gov.

DATA SYNTHESIS

We constructed evidence tables showing study, patient, and intervention characteristics; methodological quality; and outcomes, organized by KQs and CAM approach. We assessed study quality according to the criteria described in the Agency for Healthcare Research and Quality (AHRQ) *Methods Guide for Effectiveness and Comparative Effectiveness Reviews,* adapted for this review, and assigned a summary quality score of Good, Fair, or Poor to individual RCTs.

We analyzed studies to compare their characteristics, methods, and findings and compiled a summary of findings for each KQ based on qualitative and semiquantitative synthesis of the findings. There were not sufficient studies to perform quantitative meta-analyses. However, when the evidence was sufficient to estimate an effect, we computed the standardized mean difference (SMD) using Hedges g for continuous outcomes, to facilitate comparisons across studies. For each KQ, we evaluated the strength of evidence as proposed by the Grades of Recommendation, Assessment, Development, and Evaluation (GRADE) Working Group, assigning a summary rating of High, Moderate, Low, or Insufficient strength of evidence for each KQ.

PEER REVIEW

A draft version of the report was reviewed by technical experts as well as clinical leadership, and their comments are provided in the appendix.

RESULTS

We screened 1776 titles, rejected 1738, and performed a more detailed review on 38 articles. From these, we retained 7 RCTs (described in 12 articles) and 2 non-RCTs that met our eligibility criteria. Our search of www.clinicaltrials.gov yielded 438 study entries. Of these, 16 were RCTs of an eligible CAM therapy for PTSD (KQs 1–3), and 2 were non-RCTs (KQ 4).

As summarized below by KQ, most studies reviewed appeared to be preliminary investigations and were underpowered, limited by significant design flaws, and often provided inadequate descriptions of the intervention to permit replication. All studies reported short-term effects of the intervention on PTSD symptoms, but few studies reported effects on health-related quality of life, adverse effects, or retention rates. Perhaps the most striking finding overall was the relative dearth of available evidence on CAM applications for PTSD despite clear consumer interest and widespread use of these treatments. The limitations of the current evidence preclude strong conclusions about specific interventions, populations, formats, settings, appropriate treatment length or "dosing," or other refinements to the development of these approaches.

KQ 1. In adults with PTSD, are mind-body complementary and alternative medicine therapies (e.g., acupuncture, yoga, meditation) more efficacious than control for PTSD symptoms and health-related quality of life?

We identified six published RCTs that met our criteria for KQ 1: two examined meditation, one examined acupuncture, and three examined breathing/relaxation training. Our search of ClinicalTrials.gov identified 16 unpublished or ongoing studies relevant to this question.

Review and synthesis of these study findings suggest that meditation techniques are associated with moderate improvements in PTSD severity and health-related quality of life compared to usual care only (one fair-quality study) and individual psychotherapy (one poor-quality study). Both studies examined relatively brief, group therapy formats in male Veteran samples and did not conduct followup assessments beyond the active intervention period. For acupuncture (one good-quality study), change in PTSD symptoms and health-related quality of life was similar to that observed for group cognitive behavioral therapy and greater than waitlist control in a predominantly male, non-Veteran sample; treatment gains were retained at the 24-week followup. Relaxation was not associated with significant clinical improvement relative to active comparators, but 95 percent confidence intervals were broad (three poor-quality RCTs).

KQ 2. In adults with PTSD, are manipulative and body-based complementary and alternative medicine therapies (e.g., spinal manipulation, massage) more efficacious than control for PTSD symptoms and health-related quality of life?

We identified one published RCT that met eligibility criteria for KQ 2 and no unpublished or ongoing studies relevant to this question. The evidence from a single, poor-quality RCT of adjunctive, body-oriented therapy in eight women survivors of childhood sexual assault was insufficient to make meaningful conclusions.

KQ 3. In adults with PTSD, are complementary and alternative medicine therapies that are movement-based or involve energy therapies more efficacious than control for PTSD symptoms and health-related quality of life?

We did not identify any published, ongoing, or unpublished/completed RCTs of movement-based or energy therapies for PTSD.

KQ 4. For treatments evaluated in KQs 1–3 that lack randomized controlled trials, is there evidence from other study designs that suggests the potential for treatment efficacy?

Our evidence search identified two nonrandomized, prospective studies of CAM therapies for PTSD. One presented initial pilot findings of a multimodal intervention that included both CAM (hypnotherapy, guided imagery) and imaginal exposure techniques in male combat Veterans with strong sensitivities to olfactory triggers. The second study provided limited, initial information about the feasibility and potential utility of a brief CAM intervention that included instruction in relaxation skills and imagery techniques, including imaginal exposure. In sum, the published, nonrandomized studies identified by our systematic search provided little additional evidence of potential efficacy in PTSD for any of the CAM interventions of interest.

FUTURE RESEARCH

The limitations of the current evidence preclude our ability to draw strong conclusions to inform clinical practice or public policy regarding optimal use of CAM therapies for PTSD, yet the limitations in the available evidence point to numerous opportunities for future research. One of the most pertinent questions regarding CAM therapies for PTSD is, What effects might one expect of a given intervention relative to no intervention? This clinically relevant question is best addressed by a randomized clinical trial with a no-treatment (waitlist) comparator. However, study designs that withhold or delay treatment to those with PTSD may not be institutionally feasible or ethically defensible. Hence, alternative strategies merit consideration.

Another pertinent question is, To what extent might placebo or nonspecific effects account for observed clinical outcomes? This question can be hard to answer for CAM therapies, for which it may be difficult to design a sham procedure that is both truly inert and that appears sufficiently similar to the active intervention to isolate the specific effect of the intervention. The fields of surgical and psychotherapy research have long grappled with similar issues, and recommendations are available to inform these methodological challenges. Ultimately, the choice of which research strategy to employ should be determined by the key questions and by the plausibility and estimates of benefit based on prior research. For most CAM treatments, the basic efficacy question of "Can it work?" for PTSD has not been answered. Thus, randomized, placebo (or sham intervention) controlled trials, the gold standard for evaluating intervention effects, will be the most logical design for the majority of studies planned to evaluate CAM interventions. Small exploratory trials would be a logical next step for the CAM interventions that lack any studies of treatment effect.

Our systematic review identified seven RCTs and two nonrandomized studies of CAM interventions for PTSD. The term CAM encompasses a broad range of treatments—not all of which may hold the same level of promise as applications for PTSD. The absence of a strong signal pointing to any one CAM approach over others argues for investment in a set of adequately powered trials to evaluate the most promising therapies, rather than a single large trial for any one treatment. Given the current state of evidence, a two-pronged approach may be most appropriate at this stage to move the field forward. That is, a series of adequately-powered RCTs may be indicated for select CAM interventions for which there is a clear and strong preliminary signal, either based on good-quality, early empirical evidence (e.g., acupuncture), a sound theoretical rationale for efficacy in the absence of strong pilot findings (e.g., meditation), and/or promising data gleaned from the bench sciences (e.g., compelling animal models). For other CAM modalities for which the science and theory are even less well developed, such as energy therapies, more prudence is indicated, suggesting the utility of exploratory pilot studies as the appropriate next step. In addition, the efficiency and ultimate yield of future efforts may be further optimized by consensus agreement about, and concerted efforts to address, limitations identified in the current literature. Broadly, these limitations concern issues of appropriate design, outcomes, and replication strategies. There is an opportunity for strategic, well-designed studies to address the substantial gaps in evidence identified in this review.

ABBREVIATIONS TABLE

AHRQ	Agency for Healthcare Research and Quality
CAM	complementary and alternative medicine
CINAHL	Cumulative Index to Nursing and Allied Health Literature
GRADE	Grades of Recommendation, Assessment, Development, and Evaluation
KQ	key question
PILOTS	Published International Literature on Traumatic Stress
PTSD	posttraumatic stress disorder
RCT	randomized controlled trial
SMD	standardized mean difference

EVIDENCE REPORT

INTRODUCTION

Posttraumatic stress disorder (PTSD) is among the most common Axis I disorders, with an estimated lifetime prevalence in the U.S. of approximately 7 percent.[1] PTSD is often chronic and is associated with significant adverse consequences, including high rates of depression and other psychiatric comorbidities; substance abuse; suicidality; impaired social, occupational, and family functioning; decreased quality of life; and increased rates of medical morbidity, health risk behaviors, and health service use.[1-9] PTSD is the emotional disorder most frequently associated with combat and other potentially traumatic experiences that may occur during the course of military service (e.g., sexual assault, motor vehicle injury). Over 2.2 million U.S. troops have deployed in Operation Enduring Freedom and Operation Iraqi Freedom (OEF/OIF).[10] One anticipated consequence of this sustained period of military operations is the increased incidence of PTSD among Veterans. Among OEF/OIF Veterans who received Department of Veterans Affairs (VA) care between 2002 and 2008, 22 percent were diagnosed with PTSD.[11] In addition to increased mental health service use among this newest generation of Veterans, the VA has witnessed the sharpest increase in mental health service use among Vietnam-era Veterans.[12] As the VA strives to anticipate and serve the treatment needs of the Veteran population, including those returning from current Middle East conflicts as well as Veterans of previous service eras, identifying and implementing effective PTSD treatment approaches remains a critical priority.

Complementary and alternative medicine (CAM) interventions are popular among consumers and are widely employed to treat diverse physical and mental health conditions.[13] The results of a recent national survey show that nearly 38 percent of U.S. adults use CAM approaches to manage a range of physical and emotional health concerns, including pain, anxiety, and depression.[14,15] Such widely used practices deserve careful evaluation and may hold promise as either adjunctive or primary PTSD therapies. Thus, this evidence synthesis was requested by VA Research and Development to inform decisions on the need for research in this area. This report reviews the evidence for common CAM approaches for PTSD—excluding natural products such as nutritional supplements—and examines mind-body therapies, manipulative and body-based practices, and practices that are movement-based or involve energy therapies.

BACKGROUND

The current VA/Department of Defense (DoD) Clinical Practice Guideline for the Management of Posttraumatic Stress (October 2010)[16] recommends the following evidence-based, first-line therapies for PTSD: (1) trauma-focused cognitive behavioral psychotherapies, (2) stress inoculation training (SIT), and (3) pharmacotherapies. These recommendations are largely consistent with previously published practice guidelines and systematic reviews (e.g., Bisson and Andrew,[17] Foa and colleagues,[18] Institute of Medicine[19]).

Overview of Current Evidence-based PTSD Therapies

Trauma-focused psychotherapies

The category of trauma-focused psychotherapies incorporates several multicomponent, PTSD-specific interventions that share a theoretical foundation in cognitive behavioral principles. Consistent with a cognitive behavioral framework, the key components of trauma-focused psychotherapies may include *in vivo* and narrative/imaginal exposure as well as cognitive restructuring exercises. These treatments are designed to decrease emotional response through habituation and to modify maladaptive thoughts, behaviors, and emotions associated with PTSD. Most trauma-focused psychotherapy protocols combine administration of these exercises with psychoeducation and training in relaxation and anxiety-management techniques. Of note, several commonly employed relaxation techniques, such as breathing and muscle relaxation, are also consistent with CAM approaches. However, in the case of trauma-focused psychotherapies, these strategies are not hypothesized to be core mechanisms of change. Rather, they are introduced early in treatment to support the patient's later engagement in key trauma-focused elements of treatment (e.g., exposure techniques and cognitive exercises).

The most well established of the trauma-focused psychotherapies are prolonged exposure therapy, cognitive processing therapy, and eye movement desensitization and reprocessing (EMDR). Although the comparative efficacy of these interventions has not yet been established,[17] collectively the category of trauma-focused therapies has a strong empirical base. On average, 56 percent of patients who enter treatment (intent-to-treat) and 67 percent of patients who complete treatment no longer meet criteria for PTSD at posttreatment.[20] In clinical trials, trauma-focused therapies show large effects compared to waitlist control (average effect size = 1.11) and moderate effects compared to supportive therapy (average effect size = 0.82).[20]

Stress inoculation training approaches

SIT protocols for PTSD provide training in anxiety management and coping skills to "inoculate" against heightened stress responses that are presumed central to the maintenance of PTSD. SIT protocols provide a tool kit of cognitive behavioral and mind-body stress management techniques, including progressive muscle relaxation, breathing retraining, positive thinking and self-talk, assertiveness training, and thought stopping.[16] As with trauma-focused psychotherapies, several CAM techniques (e.g., release of muscle tension and breathing techniques to invoke relaxation) are common components of these interventions. However, SIT approaches (like trauma-focused psychotherapies) are theoretically grounded in cognitive behavioral theories of change and impart training in cognitive behavioral stress management techniques. Hence, for this review, and consistent with the theoretical basis of this treatment approach, SIT is considered a cognitive behavioral intervention.

Pharmacotherapies

First-line, evidence-based pharmacotherapies for PTSD include selective serotonin reuptake inhibitors (SSRIs) and serotonin norepinephrine reuptake inhibitors (SNRIs), administered as monotherapies.[16,18,21] Both SSRIs and SNRIs are presumed to improve psychobiological dysfunction believed to be characteristic of the syndrome of PTSD. Of the SSRIs, the strongest evidence base currently exists for paroxetine and sertraline, for which response rates are near 60 percent.[21,22]

Among the SNRIs, venlafaxine has the strongest support.[16] For example, one recent randomized controlled trial (RCT) found that 78 percent of patients treated with venlafaxine experienced a positive clinical response (i.e., > 30% decrease in symptom severity) although only 40 percent achieved remission.[23] In contrast to current clinical practice guideline recommendations, it should be noted that the Institute of Medicine's recent review of PTSD therapies (2007)[19] concluded that there is insufficient evidence to support the use of pharmacotherapies for PTSD. In response to this controversial recommendation, one committee member appended[19] an alternative conclusion in support of SSRIs as well as novel antipsychotics. Despite current controversies, pharmacotherapies—particularly SSRIs and SNRIs—are widely accepted as standard first-line treatment.

Limitations of Current Evidence-based PTSD Therapies

Despite mounting empirical support for the treatments summarized above and tremendous efforts within the clinical research community to refine and optimize these approaches, each is associated with limitations and potential barriers to broad dissemination and uptake. Issues of access, patient preference/acceptability, and suitability are the primary limiting factors. For example, trauma-focused psychotherapies may provoke emotional responses, and some patients may have difficulty managing these reactions, or may choose not to engage in therapies that can cause emotional (albeit short-term) discomfort. Thus, the current VA/DoD Clinical Practice Guideline recommends careful screening of patients' suitability for these modalities and recommends against their use with certain patients (e.g., those with current substance abuse, psychosis, or health problems for which intense physiological arousal is contraindicated).[16] Also, all current evidence-based psychotherapies require specialized training and frequent provider contact, which may limit their accessibility. This potential limitation is of particular relevance for patients located in areas in which clinical resources are limited (e.g., rural) and those whose schedules cannot readily accommodate frequent sessions (e.g., because of work constraints or lack of childcare). Finally, psychotherapies are typically delivered in mental health specialty clinics, which may present a barrier for those concerned about perceived stigma associated with receiving care in a mental health setting, or for those who distrust mental health providers.[24]

In contrast to psychotherapies for PTSD, pharmacotherapies generally require less frequent and shorter contact with a provider and are routinely administered in both mental health and primary care clinics. However, some patients are not amenable to pharmacological interventions,[25] and current evidence indicates that nearly 27 percent of patients will prematurely discontinue SSRIs due to treatment failure or adverse side effects, including sexual dysfunction, weight gain, and sleep disturbance.[26] Finally, existing studies suggest that medications alone are often not sufficient to relieve symptoms, and there is some evidence that men are less likely than women to benefit from pharmacological PTSD treatments.[27] Therefore, current evidence-based treatments for PTSD are not always appropriate, well-tolerated, accessible, adequate, or congruent with patient preferences.

Complementary and Alternative Medicine

CAM is commonly used to describe a wide range of therapies that are not generally considered standard components of modern medicine as practiced by physicians in the U.S. Yet, many CAM treatments, such as acupuncture, are part of traditional medical practices in other parts of the world. The National Center for Complementary and Alternative Medicine (NCCAM) in the National Institutes of Health (NIH) has proposed a classification system for CAM therapies that includes natural products (e.g., dietary supplements, herbal remedies, probiotics), mind-body medicine (e.g., meditation, yoga, acupuncture), manipulative and body-based practices (e.g., spinal manipulation, massage therapy), whole medical systems (e.g., traditional Chinese medicine, Ayurvedic medicine), and other alternative practices (e.g., light or magnet therapy, movement therapies). Although this definition and classification system is helpful, it is imperfect since some treatments, such as biofeedback, are considered conventional treatment by some experts and CAM treatment by others. For some CAM therapies, such as acupuncture, there is a growing body of scientific literature evaluating efficacy or possible mechanisms of action. However, for many CAM therapies there remains a lack of scientific evidence on efficacy, harms, indications, appropriate dosing, or mechanisms of action.

Rationale for an Evidence-based Synthesis of CAM Therapies for PTSD

CAM interventions are widely requested and used by mental health consumers including Veterans and active duty personnel; mental health–related concerns are among the most common reasons for seeking care from a CAM provider.[13-15,28,29] If efficacious, these treatments may merit consideration as either first-line or adjunctive PTSD treatments. Most CAM treatments considered in this report are noninvasive or minimally invasive; considered unlikely to result in adverse side effects; and in some cases may be more congruent with individual treatment preferences than currently recommended traditional treatment options. Numerous stakeholders have expressed strong interest in fostering the evidence base for these approaches in PTSD.[16,30] Consistent with these directives, this evidence synthesis was requested by VA Research and Development to inform decisions on the need for further research in this area. This report thus reviewed the evidence for common CAM approaches for treating PTSD.

METHODS

TOPIC DEVELOPMENT

This review was commissioned by the Department of Veterans Affairs' Evidence-based Synthesis Program. The key questions (KQs) were developed after a topic refinement process that included a preliminary review of published, peer-reviewed literature and consultations with content experts and key stakeholders in the treatment of PTSD. During this topic refinement process, selected CAM therapies were prioritized for the report; natural products (e.g., dietary supplements) were excluded. CAM therapies were classified using categories proposed by the NCCAM, and the KQs reflect this classification.

The final KQs were:

KQ 1. In adults with PTSD, are mind-body complementary and alternative medicine therapies (e.g., acupuncture, yoga, meditation) more efficacious than control for PTSD symptoms and health-related quality of life?

KQ 2. In adults with PTSD, are manipulative and body-based complementary and alternative medicine therapies (e.g., spinal manipulation, massage) more efficacious than control for PTSD symptoms and health-related quality of life?

KQ 3. In adults with PTSD, are complementary and alternative medicine therapies that are movement-based or involve energy therapies more efficacious than control for PTSD symptoms and health-related quality of life?

KQ 4. For treatments evaluated in KQs 1–3 that lack randomized controlled trials, is there evidence from other study designs that suggests the potential for treatment efficacy?

ANALYTIC FRAMEWORK

We developed and followed a standard protocol for all steps of this review. Our approach was guided by the analytic framework shown in Figure 1.

Figure 1. Analytic framework for CAM therapies for PTSD

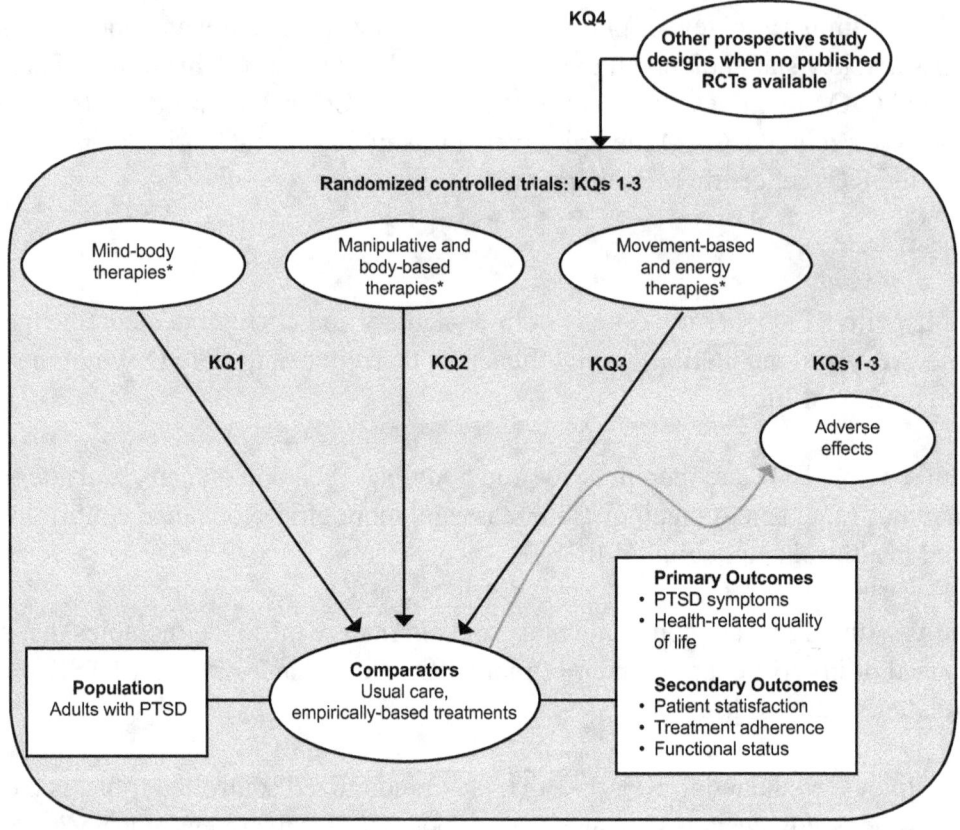

Examples of interventions:
- **Mind-body therapies:** acupuncture, meditation, yoga, deep-breathing exercises, guided imagery, hypnotherapy, progressive relaxation, and tai chi
- **Manipulative and body-based therapies:** spinal manipulation and massage therapy
- **Movement-based therapies:** Feldenkrais method, Alexander technique, Pilates, Rolfing Structural Integration, and Trager Psychophysical Integration
- **Energy therapies:** magnet therapy, light therapy, qi gong, Reiki, and healing touch

SEARCH STRATEGY

We searched English-language publications in MEDLINE® (via PubMed®), Embase®, PsycINFO®, Cumulative Index to Nursing and Allied Health Literature® (CINAHL), and the Cochrane Controlled Trials Registry from database inception through December 22, 2010. Search terms included terms for CAM therapies (acupuncture, mind-body, sensory art, yoga, reflexotherapy, musculoskeletal manipulation), PTSD, and RCTs. We used these limit terms: all adults ≥ 19 years of age, humans, and English. In addition, we searched the Published International Literature on Traumatic Stress (PILOTS) database (April 26, 2011), a specialized PTSD database maintained by the National Center for Posttraumatic Stress Disorder, to identify existing systematic reviews and studies of relaxation treatments.

We supplemented electronic searching by examining the bibliographies of included studies and review articles. When RCTs were not identified, we searched for prospective studies by adapting the sensitive "therapy filter" contained in PubMed clinical queries. To assure completeness, search strategies were developed in consultation with a master librarian. The search terms and MeSH headings for the search strategies appear in Appendix A. In addition to searching the published literature, we searched ClinicalTrials.gov (www.clinicaltrials.gov) (April 7, 2011) to identify studies in progress or completed studies that have not been published in the peer-reviewed literature.

STUDY SELECTION

Using prespecified inclusion/exclusion criteria, two reviewers assessed the list of titles and abstracts. Full-text articles identified by either reviewer as potentially relevant were retrieved for further review. Each article retrieved was reviewed by two reviewers using the eligibility criteria in Appendix B; disagreements were resolved by discussion or by a third reviewer. To be included in the evidence synthesis, a study had to (1) be an RCT, (2) compare an eligible treatment to an empirically-based treatment or to a control condition, and (3) include a sample diagnosed with PTSD. Because relaxation is often used as a placebo control in trials of psychotherapy, we further specified that relaxation interventions must be presented as an active treatment and described in sufficient detail to understand the key components. As noted earlier, studies that included relaxation training introduced within the context of a standard PTSD therapy, such as prolonged exposure or SIT, were conceptualized as non-CAM and thus ineligible for this review. In the absence of any RCT for a given treatment, we examined other prospective study designs. In response to a request from stakeholders, we categorized reasons for exclusion in a subsample of 600 studies excluded during the initial abstract review. Detailed eligibility criteria are described in Table 1.

Table 1. Summary of inclusion and exclusion criteria

Study characteristic	Inclusion criteria	Exclusion criteria
Study design	KQs 1–3: RCTs KQ 4: Other study designs when no RCTs were identified[a]	Non–English language publication Non–peer-reviewed publication
Population	Adults ≥ 19 diagnosed with PTSD using DSM criteria, validated severity measures (e.g., PTSD checklist), or clinical diagnosis Patients in acute-phase treatment (i.e., not selected for treatment-resistant PTSD)	Patients with complicated PTSD or acute suicidality Studies with eligibility criteria requiring a diagnosis of PTSD comorbid with another mental or physical illness (e.g., PTSD and substance abuse)

Study characteristic	Inclusion criteria	Exclusion criteria
Interventions	Any of the following eligible treatments: • Mind-body therapies: acupuncture, meditation, yoga, deep-breathing exercises, guided imagery, hypnotherapy, progressive relaxation, and tai chi • Manipulative and body-based therapies: spinal manipulation and massage therapy • Movement-based therapies: Feldenkrais method, Alexander technique, Pilates, Rolfing Structural Integration, and Trager Psychophysical Integration • Energy therapies: magnet therapy, light therapy, qi gong, Reiki, and healing touch	Interventions used in a continuation or maintenance phase Dietary supplements Standard psychotherapies (e.g., prolonged exposure) and extensions of these therapies (e.g., mindfulness-based cognitive therapy) Relaxation used as a control arm or reported without describing the key components Biofeedback
Comparators	Studies comparing an eligible treatment to a control condition such as usual care (including no treatment), supportive therapy, attention control, sham intervention, or a waitlist Studies comparing an eligible treatment to an empirically based treatment, prolonged exposure, cognitive processing therapy, or antidepressant medication	None
Outcomes	Change in level of PTSD symptoms (i.e., on self-report and/or clinician-administered measures, including remission rates) or change in quality of life (i.e., functional status and health-related quality of life) Social functioning, patient satisfaction with treatment, treatment adherence/retention (e.g., proportion of prescribed sessions that are completed, completion of between-session assignments), and adverse treatment effects Reported at ≥ 6 weeks after treatment initiation	None
Setting	Patients recruited from community or outpatient mental health or general medical settings	Studies conducted outside North America, Western Europe, Australia, or New Zealand. Studies conducted outside of these countries were unlikely to be applicable to VA populations because of important differences in culture and health care systems.

[a]The eligibility criteria for nonrandomized controlled trials matched the criteria for KQs 1–3 except for study design. For each intervention that lacked eligible RCTs, we included prospective studies (nonrandomized controlled trials, controlled before-and-after studies, and prospective cohort studies and case series).

Abbreviations: DSM = Diagnostic and Statistical Manual of Mental Disorders, PTSD = posttraumatic stress disorder, RCT = randomized controlled trial, VA = Veterans Affairs

Studies identified from the ClinicalTrials.gov search were included if they were an RCT of an eligible CAM intervention and evaluated adults with PTSD. In addition, we included completed studies when a MEDLINE search (April 2011) using the name of the principal investigator did not identify a published study reporting clinical outcomes.

DATA ABSTRACTION

A trained researcher abstracted data from published reports into a data abstraction form (Appendix C); a second reviewer overread the abstracted data. We resolved disagreements by consensus among the first and second reviewer or by obtaining a third reviewer's opinion when consensus could not be reached. We abstracted the following data for each included study:

- study design
- setting
- population characteristics
- subject eligibility and exclusion criteria
- number of subjects and providers
- intervention(s)
- comparison(s)
- length of followup
- outcome(s)

For studies identified in ClinicalTrials.gov with no identified peer-reviewed publication of study results, we abstracted a limited set of data: study title, intervention, comparator, funding agency, funding dates, and study status.

QUALITY ASSESSMENT

We assessed the risk of bias pertaining to the key questions using the quality criteria described in the Agency for Healthcare Research and Quality (AHRQ) *Methods Guide for Effectiveness and Comparative Effectiveness Reviews* (hereafter referred to as the *Methods Guide*),[31] adapted for this specific topic. For RCTs, we abstracted data on adequacy of randomization and allocation concealment, comparability of groups at baseline, blinding, completeness of followup and differential loss to followup, whether incomplete data were addressed appropriately, validity of outcome measures and completeness of outcomes reporting, and conflict of interest. Using these data elements, we assigned a summary quality score of Good, Fair, or Poor to individual RCTs. Because non-RCT studies were included for descriptive purposes, we did not assess their quality.

We assessed studies for applicability to U.S. Veterans. In addition to the quality rating for individual studies, we evaluated the overall quality of the evidence for each KQ as proposed by the Grades of Recommendation, Assessment, Development, and Evaluation (GRADE) Working Group (Appendix D).[32]

DATA SYNTHESIS

We critically analyzed studies to compare their characteristics, methods, and findings. We compiled a summary of findings for each KQ or clinical topic and drew conclusions based on a qualitative synthesis of the findings. There were not sufficient studies to perform quantitative meta-analyses. When the evidence was sufficient to estimate an effect, we computed the standardized mean difference (SMD) using Hedges g for continuous outcomes, to facilitate comparisons across studies. The SMD is useful when studies assess the same outcome, but with different measures. In this circumstance, it is necessary to standardize the results for the studies to a uniform scale to facilitate comparisons and to combine in meta-analysis. We calculated the SMD for each study by subtracting (at posttest) the average score of the control group from the average score of the experimental group and dividing the result by the pooled standard deviations (SDs) of the experimental and control groups. A negative SMD indicates a greater effect in the intervention group. For example, an effect size of -0.5 indicates that the mean decline in PTSD symptom severity for the experimental group is half an SD greater than the mean decline in the control group. SMD is commonly interpreted as small (0.2), moderate (0.5), or large (≥ 0.80).[33,34]

RATING THE BODY OF EVIDENCE

We assessed the overall body of evidence for outcomes using a method developed by the GRADE Working Group, which classified the grade of evidence across outcomes according to the following criteria:

- High—Further research is very unlikely to change our confidence on the estimate of effect.
- Moderate—Further research is likely to have an important impact on our confidence in the estimate of effect and may change the estimate.
- Low—Further research is very likely to have an important impact on our confidence in the estimate of effect and is likely to change the estimate.
- Insufficient—Evidence on an outcome is absent or too weak, sparse, or inconsistent to estimate an effect.

PEER REVIEW

A draft version of the report was reviewed by technical experts and clinical leadership, and their comments are provided in Appendix E.

RESULTS

LITERATURE SEARCH

We identified 1776 unique citations from a combined search of MEDLINE® (via PubMed®, n = 353), Embase® (n = 451), CINAHL® (n = 429), PsychINFO® (n = 390), Cochrane Database of Systematic Reviews (n = 32), and the PILOTS database (n = 121). By manual examination of the bibliographies of included studies and review articles, we identified four additional citations. Of these, 1738 were excluded at the title-and-abstract level. Of the 1738 studies excluded at the title-and-abstract level, we reevaluated and categorized the reason for exclusion in a subsample of 600 citations. The most common reasons for exclusion were review article (23%); a drug or a non-CAM intervention (22%); a "standard treatment" (e.g., EMDR or CBT) without a CAM comparator (14%); a sample under 19 years of age (13%); a sample that did not have PTSD (10%); and evaluation of therapies that were neither standard for PTSD nor for CAM (10%).

An additional 29 studies were excluded following full-text review. The question of what type of relaxation study was applicable to our report was a complicated one. Our literature search identified six citations that included a relaxation treatment arm but did not meet full eligibility criteria. Of these, one did not evaluate a population with PTSD;[35] one was determined not to be CAM because the relaxation was delivered in conjunction with biofeedback;[36] two conceptualized the relaxation as a control group rather than an active treatment;[37,38] and one study with three citations did not describe the key components of the relaxation intervention such that it could not be categorized as CAM or otherwise.[39-41]

Nine published studies were retained and abstracted for this evidence synthesis, including 7 RCTs (described in 12 articles) and 2 non-RCTs. Five articles contained previously described demographic or descriptive data for the seven RCTs; these studies are referred to as "companion" studies.

Additionally, our search of www.clinicaltrials.gov identified 438 potentially relevant, unpublished trials. Of these, 16 were RCTs of an eligible CAM therapy for PTSD and are described in the applicable KQ sections that follow. There were also three non-RCTs, described in the KQ 4 section.

Figure 2 illustrates each step of our literature search process. Appendix F provides a complete listing of articles excluded at the full-text stage, with reasons for exclusion.

Figure 2. Literature flow diagram

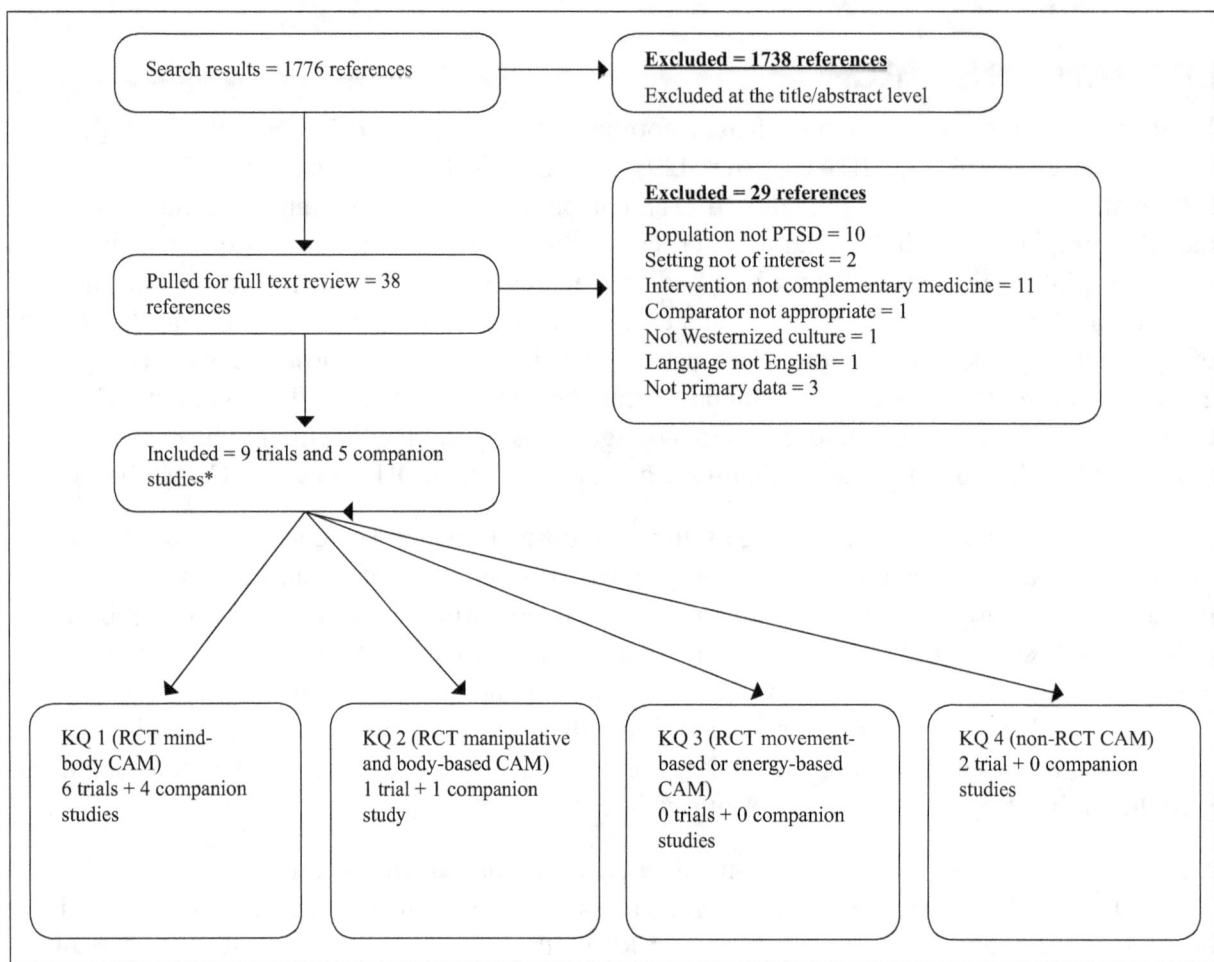

*Reference list includes additional references cited for background and methods plus Web sites relevant to KQs.

Abbreviations: KQ = key question, CAM = complementary and alternative medicine, PTSD = posttraumatic stress disorder, RCT = randomized controlled trial

STUDY CHARACTERISTICS

Basic characteristics of these studies are summarized in Table 2. A total of 7 RCTs (296 subjects) and 2 non-RCTs (41 subjects) met eligibility criteria. Of the RCTs, three evaluated relaxation, two evaluated meditation, and one each evaluated acupuncture and massage interventions. There were no RCTs identified that examined movement-based or energy therapies. To be eligible for participation, all studies required patients to meet DSM criteria for PTSD, and four of the seven RCTs included military Veterans. All studies reported PTSD symptom outcomes, but health-related quality of life (HRQOL), patient satisfaction, social functioning, and adverse effects were reported less frequently. Only one RCT was good quality.

Common study limitations included (1) a lack of power to draw meaningful conclusions, (2) the absence of explanations for missing data and dropouts, and (3) analyses that were performed on completers rather than intent-to-treat samples. In addition, important aspects of the study design and sample characteristics were frequently unclear in the fair- and poor-quality articles. For example, it was difficult in every case to discern whether the groups being compared were truly comparable at baseline. The nonrandomized studies used prospective cohort and case series designs.

Table 2. Summary of study characteristics

Study	Study design (n)	Quality[a]	Intervention vs. comparator	Outcome measures[b]
RCTs of mind-body interventions: KQ 1				
Bormann et al., 2008[42]	RCT (n = 29)	Fair	Mantram repetition vs. usual care	CAPS, PCL, Q-LES-Q-SF, FACIT-SpEx4, CSQ
Brooks and Scarano, 1985[43]	RCT (n = 25)	Poor	Transcendental meditation vs. psychotherapy	PVSDS, individual items to assess employment status and family problems
Echeburúa et al., 1996[44]	RCT (n = 20)	Poor	Progressive muscle relaxation vs. cognitive behavioral therapy	SS-PTSD, SOA
Hollifield et al, 2007[45]	RCT (n = 84)	Good	Acupuncture vs. group cognitive behavioral therapy vs. waitlist	PSS-SR, SDI
Vaughan et al., 1994[46]	RCT (n = 36)	Fair	Applied muscle relaxation vs. image habituation training vs. EMDR	SI-PTSD, IES
Watson et al., 1997[47]	RCT (n = 90)	Poor	Simple relaxation instruction vs. relaxation instruction + deep breathing vs. relaxation instruction + deep breathing and thermal biofeedback	PTSD-I M-PTSD
RCT of manipulative and body-based interventions: KQ 2				
Price, 2006[48,49]	RCT (n = 8)	Poor	Body-oriented therapy (massage) vs. waitlist	CR-PTSD
Non-RCTs of CAM therapies for PTSD: KQ 4				
Abramowitz and Lichtenberg, 2010[50]	Prospective cohort (n = 36)	NA	Hypnotherapeutic olfactory conditioning	IES-R
Hossack and Bentall, 1996[51]	Case series (n = 5); 17 and 29 weeks	NA	Relaxation and visual kinesthetic dissociation	IES

[a]Study quality assessed via key quality criteria described in Agency for Healthcare Research and Quality's (AHRQ's) *Methods Guide for Effectiveness and Comparative Effectiveness Reviews.*[31]

[b]Outcomes limited to those with direct relevance to KQs 1–4 (i.e., PTSD severity/diagnosis, HRQOL).

Abbreviations: CAPS = Clinician-Administered PTSD Scale, CR-PTSD = Crime-Related Post Traumatic Stress Disorder Scale, EMDR = eye movement desensitization and reprocessing, FACIT-SpEx4 = Functional Assessment of Chronic Illness Therapy–Spirituality-Expanded Version 4, IES = Impact of Events Scale, IES-R = Impact of Events Scale–Revised, M-PTSD = Mississippi Scale for Combat-Related PTSD, NA = not applicable, PCL = Posttraumatic Stress Disorder Checklist (-M is military version), PSS-SR = Posttraumatic Symptom Scale–Self Report, PTSD-I = Posttraumatic Stress Disorder Interview, PVSDS = Post-Vietnam Stress Disorder Scale, Q-LES-Q-SF = Quality of Life Enjoyment and Satisfaction Questionnaire–Short Form, RCT = randomized controlled trial, SI-PTSD = PTSD Structured Interview, SOA = Scale of Adaptation, SS-PTSD = Scale of Severity of Posttraumatic Stress Disorder, SDI = Sheehan Disability Inventory

Table 3 summarizes the outcome measures included in this evidence synthesis, listing the abbreviated and full name of each instrument, format, number of items, score range, and interpretation of scoring.

Table 3. Summary of outcome measures

Abbreviation	Name of instrument	Format	# of items	Range	Interpretation
CAPS[a]	Clinician-Administered PTSD Scale	Semistructured interview	17	0–136	Higher score = more severe PTSD symptoms
CR-PTSD[b]	Crime-Related Post Traumatic Stress Disorder Scale	Self-report scale	28	0–112	Higher score = more severe PTSD symptoms
CSQ	Client Satisfaction Questionnaire	Self-report scale	8	8–36	Higher score = more satisfaction with treatment
FACIT-SpEx4	Functional Assessment of Chronic Illness Therapy–Spirituality-Expanded Version 4	Self-report scale	23	0–184	Higher score = better quality of life
IES[c]	Impact of Events Scale	Self-report scale	15	0–75	Higher score = more severe PTSD symptoms
IES-R	Impact of Events Scale–Revised	Self-report scale	22	0–88	Higher score = more severe PTSD symptoms
M-PTSD	Mississippi Scale for Combat-Related PTSD	Self-report scale	35	35–175	Higher score = more severe PTSD symptoms
PCL	PTSD Checklist	Self-report scale	17	17–85	Higher score = more severe PTSD symptoms
PSS-SR	Posttraumatic Symptom Scale–Self-Report	Self-report scale	17	0–51	Higher score = more severe PTSD symptoms
PTSD-I	Posttraumatic Stress Disorder Interview	Structured interview	17	17–119	Higher score = more severe PTSD symptoms
PVSDS	Post-Vietnam Stress Disorder Scale (unpublished)	NR	NR	NR	Higher score = more severe PTSD symptoms
Q-LES-Q-SF	Quality of Life Enjoyment and Satisfaction–Short Form	Self-report scale	14	14–70	Higher score = better quality of life
SDI	Sheehan Disability Inventory	Self-report scale	3	0–30	Higher score = greater functional impairment
SI-PTSD	PTSD Structured Interview	Structured interview	17	0–68	Higher score = more severe PTSD symptoms
SOA	Scale of Adaptation	Self-report scale	6	6–36	Lower score = better adaption to impact of sexual aggression on daily life
SS-PTSDS	Scale of Severity of Posttraumatic Stress Disorder Symptoms	Structured interview	51	0–51	Higher score = more severe PTSD symptoms

[a]Numerous scoring strategies exist. The number of items/range of scores presented here refer only to the interview items that assess DSM-IV diagnostic criteria. Additional CAPS items may administered to assess functioning, response validity, and presence of associated symptoms.

[b]Score is typically calculated and interpreted as the average item score.

[c]The IES does not assess Cluster D/hyperarousal PTSD symptoms, whereas the IES-R does include items to assess this symptom cluster.

Abbreviations: NR = not reported, PTSD = posttraumatic stress disorder

KEY QUESTION 1: In adults with PTSD, are mind-body complementary and alternative medicine therapies (e.g., acupuncture, yoga, meditation) more efficacious than control for PTSD symptoms and health-related quality of life?

Published literature

We identified six published RCTs that met our criteria for KQ 1. Of these, two examined meditation,[42,43] one examined acupuncture,[45] and three examined breathing/relaxation training.[44,46,47] These studies are summarized in Table 4 and discussed in this section.

In addition to the published literature, our search of ClinicalTrials.gov identified 16 unpublished or ongoing studies relevant to this question (Table 5).

Table 4. Characteristics of mind-body interventions (KQ 1)

Study and quality rating	Population	Design details	Intervention	Comparator	Outcomes[a]
Bormann et al., 2008[42] Fair	N = 29 Trauma: combat Mean age (SD): 56 (6.57) Male: 29 (100%) Military Veterans: 29 (100%)	PTSD diagnosis: DSM-IV by CAPS Key exclusions: Psychotic disorder Severe suicidality Inability to participate in a group Recruitment: PTSD orientation groups, fliers, brochures	6 weekly, 90-minute group sessions of mantram repetition + home practice Led by psychiatric nurses	Usual care	Remission: NR Response: ES = between group differences NR HRQOL: ES = between group differences NR AE: NR Followup duration: 6 weeks (end of treatment)
Brooks and Scarano, 1985[43] Poor	N = 25 Trauma: combat Mean age (SD): 33.3 (NR) Male: 25 (100%) Military Veterans: 25 (100%)	PTSD diagnosis: DSM-III (means of assessment not specified) Key exclusions: Substance abuse Major tranquilizers Psychiatric hospitalization Suicidal or homicidal Currently practicing TM Recruitment: from mental health clinic	4-day workshop on transcendental meditation (TM), then weekly 60-minute sessions for 11 weeks + home practice 20 minutes/day, twice daily) Led by Maharishi-trained leader	Individual psychotherapy	Remission: NR Response: decreased PTSD symptom severity, p < .05; emotional numbness, p < .025 HRQOL: decreased family problems, p < .05 AE: NR Followup duration: 12 weeks (end of treatment)
Echeburúa et al., 1996[44] Poor	N = 20 Trauma: rape/sex assault Mean age (SD): 22 (6.9) Women: 20 (100%) Veterans: none	PTSD diagnosis: DSM-IIIR by SS-PTSDS Key exclusions: Other serious mental illness Time since trauma > 3 months Recruitment: Consecutive patients seeking treatment	Progressive muscle relaxation (PMR) Five 1-hour sessions Intervention not well described	Cognitive restructuring, coping skills training, and PMR	Remission: 5 of 10 treatments vs. 8 of 10 control had no symptoms Response: no between group differences HRQOL: NR AE: NR Followup duration: 5 weeks (end of treatment) and 2,4,7, 13 months

Study and quality rating	Population	Design details	Intervention	Comparator	Outcomes[a]
Hollifield et al., 2007[45] Good	N = 84 Trauma: childhood sexual/ physical abuse Mean age (SD) 42.2 (NR) Male: 27 (32.14%) Veterans: none	PTSD diagnosis: DSM-IV by SCID Key exclusions: substance abuse, psychosis, current other active treatment for PTSD Recruitment: clinical referral, advertisement, flyers, other media, professional contacts, word of mouth	Acupuncture (traditional Chinese medicine) with 11 to 14 solid needles placed for 25–40 minutes with manipulation + 15 minutes/day of home-based therapy (ear seeds)	Cognitive behavioral therapy or waitlist	Remission: NR Response (PSS-SR < 16): Acupuncture = 15 (63%), maintained at 24 weeks CBT = 9 (36%), increased to 13 (52%) at 24 weeks Waitlist = 4 (17%), NR at 24 weeks HRQOL: acupuncture and CBT groups improved compared to WL control AE: 1 in acupuncture group Followup duration: 12 weeks (end of treatment) and 24 weeks
Vaughan et al., 1994[46] Fair	N = 36 Trauma: childhood abuse, sexual/physical assault, transportation Mean age (SD): 32 (14.7) Male: 13 (36.11%) Veterans: none	PTSD diagnosis: DSM-IIIR by SI-PTSD Key exclusions: severe personality disorder, psychosis Recruitment: from mental health clinic	Applied muscle relaxation (early recognition of anxiety, progressive muscle relaxation, passive muscle ("release-only") relaxation, cue-controlled relaxation	EMDR or exposure therapy	Remission: no between group differences Response: no between group differences HRQOL: NR AE: NR Followup duration: 2 to 3 weeks (end of treatment) and 24 weeks
Watson et al., 1997[47] Poor	N = 90 Trauma: combat Mean age (SD): 45.6 (NR) Male: 90 (100%) Military Veterans: 90 (100%)	PTSD diagnosis: DSM-IIIR by PTSD-I Key exclusions: NR Recruitment: NR	10 weekly, 30-minute sessions of relaxation instruction (RI) or RI + deep breathing instruction	10, weekly, 30-minute sessions of RI, deep breathing + thermal biofeedback	Remission: NR Response: NR HRQOL: NR AE: NR Followup duration: NR

[a]If comparator, outcomes given for intervention versus comparator.

Abbreviations: AE = adverse effects, CAPS = Clinician-Administered PTSD Scale, DSM = Diagnostic and Statistical Manual, EMDR = eye movement desensitization and reprocessing, ES = effect size, HRQOL = health-related quality of life, PCL = PTSD Checklist, PSS-SR = Posttraumatic Symptom Scale–Self Report, PTSD-I = Post-traumatic Stress Disorder Interview. Q-LES-Q-SF = Quality of Life Enjoyment and Satisfaction Questionnaire–Short Form, NR = not reported, NS = not significant, RI = relaxation instruction, SCID = Structured Clinical Interview for DSM, SD = standard deviation, SI-PTSD = PTSD Structured Interview

Meditation

Although various typologies of meditation practice exist, meditation may be broadly classified as concentrative or nonconcentrative (e.g., mindfulness meditation), depending on the manner in which mental attention is entrained. Concentrative techniques are those in which the practitioner intensely focuses on a particular object (e.g., a candle flame, the sensation of breathing, a word or sound) and tries to repeatedly bring focus back to the object if attention falters. In contrast, nonconcentrative techniques encourage practitioners to cultivate awareness and acceptance of all mental events. The goal is to observe moment-to-moment shifts in one's internal experiences without controlling or judging their content.

In this evidence synthesis, we identified two studies[42,43] involving a total of 54 patients that compared concentrative meditation to control (1 study) or to an active comparator (1 study). Both studies enrolled samples of male combat Veterans into group-based interventions and encouraged regular home practice. Sample sizes were relatively modest (n = 25 to 29), treatment length was brief (6 to 12 weeks), and outcomes were assessed at posttreatment only. We did not identify any published studies of nonconcentrative meditative techniques for PTSD.

Bormann and colleagues (2008)[42] conducted a fair-quality RCT of 29 male combat Veterans who met DSM-IV criteria for PTSD. Participants were recruited from a VA medical center via clinical orientation groups or flyers and brochures. Participants randomized to the mantram intervention received six, 90-minute, weekly group sessions co-led by two psychiatric nurses. Session content included the use of mantram repetition (i.e., the spiritual practice of repeating a sacred word or phrase) to manage PTSD symptoms, slow down thinking to decrease reactivity, and foster mindfulness to train attention. Home practice and self-monitoring were encouraged. Participants randomized to this condition were allowed to maintain usual care, including medications. Patients allocated to the control condition received "usual care" that was not described further. Key inclusion criteria were male VA participants diagnosed with combat-related PTSD. Those with current psychosis or severe suicidality or those deemed unable to participate in a group were excluded.

Outcomes were assessed at posttreatment (6 weeks). PTSD severity was assessed with the Clinician-Administered PTSD Scale (CAPS) and PTSD checklist (PCL). HRQOL was assessed with the Functional Assessment of Chronic Illness Therapy–Spirituality-Expanded Version 4 (FACIT-SpEx4) and Quality of Life Enjoyment and Satisfaction Questionnaire–Short Form (Q-LES-Q-SF). Satisfaction with the mantram intervention was assessed with the Client Satisfaction Questionnaire (CSQ). Adverse effects and treatment adherence (i.e., group session adherence, home practice) were not reported. Steps to ensure treatment fidelity included the use of a treatment manual and expert review of randomly selected session recordings. This trial was conceptualized as a feasibility study, and some of its limitations were consistent with a preliminary effort, including nonblinding of group assignment, failure to report or address missing data, and a lack of followup assessments. In addition, the authors did not report or account for potential baseline between-group differences (e.g., PTSD severity) that may have influenced the findings.

Participants were randomized to the mantram intervention (n = 14) or control (n = 15). Change scores and effect sizes were provided for all outcome measures. However, because no inferential analyses were conducted, the statistical significance of reported differences was unclear. Posttreatment decreases in the severity of PTSD symptoms were larger in the intervention group compared to control. For the CAPS, mean change was -4.79 (SD = 7.45) versus -2.64 (SD = 5.44); effect size: -0.33. For the PCL, mean change was -8.79 (SD = 12.64) versus -1.20 (SD = 7.95); effect size: -0.72. A similar pattern of improvement was observed on both measures of HRQOL. For the Q-LES-Q-SF, mean change was 0.64 (SD = 0.93) versus 0.07 (SD = 0.70); effect size: 0.70. For the FACIT-SpEx4, mean change was 10.14 (SD = 9.49) versus 2.64 (SD = 12.62); effect size: 0.67. Eighty-six percent of participants who completed the mantram intervention, including those initially randomized to the waitlist control, rated their treatment satisfaction as "moderate to high" on the CSQ (mean scores not provided).

Brooks and Scarano (1985)[43] conducted a poor-quality RCT that allocated 25 patients to either a 12-week transcendental meditation (TM) group (n = 13) or individual psychotherapy (n = 12). TM is a spiritually-based form of mantram. All potential participants were seeking treatment for combat-related trauma symptoms at the Denver Vet Center. No specific inclusion criteria were listed, and it was not clear if all participants met full diagnostic criteria for PTSD. Exclusion criteria included history of psychiatric hospitalization, current suicidal or homicidal ideation, or currently practicing TM. With the exception of the study treatments, the authors did not specify whether participants were able to begin or continue other behavioral or pharmacological therapies during the study period.

TM was taught in a 4-day workshop that included daily 90-minute sessions led by an individual who was trained by Maharishi Mahesh Yogi (TM developer), followed by 11, 1-hour, weekly followup meetings. Home practice for 20 minutes twice daily was recommended. No additional information about the TM trainer was provided. Therapists providing psychotherapy to participants randomized to the comparison condition held a minimum of a master's degree in social work or psychology. The primary study outcomes, measured at baseline and posttreatment (12 weeks), were the "degree" of PTSD and emotional numbness assessed with the Post-Vietnam Stress Disorder Scale (PVSDS), an unpublished measure. Additional items assessed aspects of HRQOL, including employment status and family problems. Adverse effects (except for discontinuation) were not reported.

Several significant design flaws limited interpretability of study findings, including the use of unpublished and unvalidated measures; failure to describe subject characteristics (although the authors indicated that there were no between-group differences at baseline); no measure of adherence (group attendance, home practice) or treatment fidelity; and failure to measure or report other treatments received during the study period. Because a single interventionist delivered the TM intervention, treatment and therapist effects were confounded. Finally, although not specifically addressed by the authors, this preliminary study enrolled a relatively modest sample size and certainly was not adequately powered for equivalence hypothesis testing (nor was it intended to be).

Comparable proportions of participants in each study arm completed 12 weeks of treatment: 10 (77%) completed TM and 8 (67%) completed individual therapy. Reasons for discontinuation were not reported. Mean pretreatment and posttreatment scores were provided for the PVSDS. However, no information was provided about possible range and interpretation of scores, which largely limited their interpretability. Controlling for pretreatment values, greater reduction in PTSD severity was observed for the TM group (9.70 ± 2.98 to 5.80 ± 4.26) versus psychotherapy group (11.71 ± 2.63 to 10.86 ± 2.85, $p < .05$). This was also true for the Emotional Numbness Scale for

TM versus psychotherapy (3.70 ± 1.64 to 1.70 ± 1.95 versus 3.75 ± 1.03 to 3.50 ± 1.41, $p < 0.05$, respectively). At posttreatment, those in the TM group were also more likely to report fewer family problems ($p < 0.05$), whereas no between-group difference in employment status was observed. Within-group, paired t-tests showed significant improvement on all self-reported measures for the TM group and no significant changes at posttreatment for the psychotherapy group.

To summarize, the findings of two short-term RCTs provided limited support for two forms of concentrative meditation for combat-related PTSD. Both studies examined relatively brief group therapy formats in all-male Veteran samples, with demonstrated effects on PTSD severity and HRQOL. However, both were preliminary inquiries, and design limitations compromised interpretability and generalizability of reported findings. Yet, together these studies demonstrate the feasibility of enrolling and retaining male Veterans into meditation group interventions, and both recorded improvement in posttreatment symptoms relative to baseline levels.

Acupuncture

Acupuncture, a branch of traditional Chinese medicine, has been used to treat mental illness in other countries for centuries. It comprises a varied group of procedures that can include needle placement in preselected or individually chosen points; in subcutaneous tissue or muscle; with or without manipulation, electrical stimulation or the use of "ear seeds" in addition to needle placement. However, it is unknown whether acupuncture can be used to treat PTSD successfully.

We identified a single, good-quality RCT by Hollifield and colleagues (2007)[45] that allocated 84 patients who met DSM-IV criteria for PTSD either to acupuncture (n = 29); cognitive behavioral therapy (CBT) sessions (n = 28); or a waitlist control (n = 27). The intervention period was 12 weeks and comprised 24 acupuncture sessions or weekly group CBT sessions. Participants in the study were recruited by clinician referrals and advertisements in the local media; no VA or DoD settings were included. Key exclusions were comorbid psychotic disorder or substance abuse or current engagement in a PTSD-specific treatment. However, participants could continue stable supportive therapy or prescribed medication for another psychiatric disorder, such as depression.

Biweekly acupuncture treatments were 60 minutes each and included a symptom interview; pulse and tongue evaluation; needle insertion, manipulation, and retention; and Vaccaria seed (or "ear seed") placement. Participants were instructed to massage the seeds, which were taped to specific points on the ear, for 15 minutes every day between sessions. Treatment was administered by an experienced, licensed acupuncturist trained in traditional Chinese medicine. Weekly, 2-hour group CBT sessions followed a manualized protocol. To equalize amount of attention to the problem the two groups experienced, home practice of CBT methods for 15 minutes/day was also encouraged, but adherence was not measured. The training and experience level of the therapist who led the CBT groups were not specified. Only one interventionist was assigned to each intervention; thus, treatment and therapist effects were confounded.

Assessments were conducted at baseline, 12 weeks (end of treatment), and 6 months (3-month followup). PTSD severity was measured with the Posttraumatic Symptom Scale–Self Report (PSS-SR), and HRQOL was measured with the Sheehan Disability Inventory (SDI). Treatment satisfaction was assessed among those randomized to acupuncture or CBT with a 10-item scale developed by the authors ($\alpha = 0.87$). Neither treatment adherence nor treatment fidelity was reported. Among the 29 participants randomized to acupuncture, 65.5 percent were retained. Five withdrew before initiation of treatment and thus were not included in the analyzed sample (i.e., no baseline data). An additional five participants withdrew during treatment for the following reasons: incarceration (n = 1); conflicting medical treatments (n = 2); perceived adverse effects of acupuncture (n = 1); and difficulty keeping appointments (n = 1). Of the 28 participants randomized to CBT, 75 percent were retained. Three withdrew before treatment, and 4 withdrew during treatment due to difficulty keeping appointments (n = 2) and unknown reasons (n = 2). Among the 27 participants randomized to waitlist control, 77.8 percent were retained. Three withdrew before treatment, and three withdrew during the study period for unstated reasons. Intent-to-treat analyses included all participants for whom baseline data were available: acupuncture (n = 24); CBT (n = 25); and waitlist control (n = 24). Missing data were estimated using the last-observation-carried-forward method.

Mean PSS-SR scores decreased from baseline to the 12-week assessment in both the acupuncture group (31.3 ± 10.1 to 15.6 ± 13.9) and CBT group (32.5 ± 6.6 to 20.0 ± 10.6; $p < .05$) but remained essentially unchanged in the waitlist group (30.8 ± 9.5 to 27.9 ± 12.3). At 6 months, the treatment effects on PTSD symptoms persisted (PSS-SR scores =15.4, acupuncture; 16.7, CBT; and 27.9, waitlist control). Pairwise contrasts from 0 to 12 weeks were not statistically different between acupuncture and CBT ($p = 0.29$). Pairwise contrasts were statistically significant between both waitlist and acupuncture ($p < 0.01$) and CBT ($p < 0.01$).

Similar findings were observed for all three study arms on the SDI: scores decreased from baseline to the 12-week assessment in both acupuncture (3.8 ± 0.8 to 3.0 ± 1.3) and CBT (4.1 ± 0.8 to 3.3 ± 1.2; $p < .05$) but were again essentially unchanged in the waitlist control. SDI scores remained relatively stable across all three groups at 6 months. As with the PSS-SR, pairwise contrasts from baseline to posttreatment for the SDI were not statistically different between acupuncture and CBT ($p = .83$); However, there were statistically significant differences between waitlist and both acupuncture ($p = .01$) and CBT($p < .01$). Global satisfaction with care was high, and there was no significant difference between groups in both acupuncture and CBT.

In summary, the findings from a single, good-quality RCT suggested that a 12-week course of acupuncture treatments was similar to group CBT (although not powered for equivalence hypothesis testing) and more effective than no acupuncture in reducing PTSD symptoms and improving HRQOL. The clinical improvement associated with acupuncture or CBT persisted for at least 3 months after completion of treatment.

Relaxation

Three studies involving 146 patients[44,46,47] compared forms of relaxation training to active comparators; one also included a third, attention control arm[47] Study quality ranged from poor[44,47] to fair.[46]

The RCT by Echeburúa and colleagues (1996)[44] randomly assigned 20 women who had experienced sexual aggression in the past 3 months to a CBT-based intervention that included cognitive restructuring plus coping skills training and progressive muscle relaxation (PMR)—or to PMR alone. In this comparative effectiveness design, both interventions consisted of five, 60-minute, weekly sessions administered by a doctoral-level therapist with 5 years' experience conducting CBT for sexual assault-related PTSD. The therapist also was responsible for conducting all study assessments. Participants were recruited from three psychological counseling centers for women in Spain. All met DSM-IIIR criteria for acute PTSD (i.e., symptoms had persisted for > 1 month and < 3 months) per the Scale of Severity of Posttraumatic Stress Disorder Symptoms (SS-PTSDS). Severe psychiatric comorbidity (e.g., schizophrenia, mental deficiency) was the primary exclusion criteria.

The cognitive restructuring plus specific coping skills training intervention included:

- psychoeducation about sexual trauma and PTSD
- introduction of CBT techniques for modifying maladaptive thoughts and feelings related to sexual trauma
- coping skills training including PMR, thought stopping, and distraction
- instructions for self-guided exposure to avoided situations and stimuli

The PMR alone intervention provided psychoeducation and training in progressive muscle relaxation. For both conditions, PMR followed methods proposed by Bernstein and Borkovec.[52] This study was considered poor quality because of nonblinding of subjects or the assessor/ therapist, unclear randomization and allocation concealment, and no intent-to-treat analysis. Power was not calculated a priori and clearly was inadequate for comparative analyses. There was no measure of treatment fidelity, and adherence was unclear. Finally, inclusion of PMR in both intervention arms complicated interpretation of study findings in the absence of a clearer description of how applying this technique may have differed between treatment conditions.

Outcomes were assessed at baseline; posttreatment (5 weeks after baseline); and at approximately 2, 4, 7, and 13 months after baseline (i.e., 1, 3, 6, and 12 months after the end of treatment). It appears that all 20 patients completed treatment and remained in the study through the 13-month assessment. At baseline, mean score on the SS-PTSDS, the primary outcome measure, was 35.5 (SD = 7.96). Within groups, mean scores decreased from baseline to posttreatment, from 36.7 (SD = 8.59) to 12 (SD = 6.94) for the cognitive restructuring plus coping skills group, and from 34.3 (SD = 7.54) to 18.7 (SD = 9.20) for the PMR group. Scores decreased slightly in subsequent assessments in both groups. There were no statistically significant between-group differences. At posttreatment, 8 out of 10 patients (80%) in the cognitive restructuring plus coping skills group and 5 out of 10 (50%) in the PMR group no longer met criteria for PTSD. Additional improvements were observed at the 2-month followup (100% remission in the cognitive restructuring plus coping skills group versus 80% remission in the PMR group), which were retained at the 13-month followup. Results of the Scale of Adaptation (SOA), a measure of functional adaptation to the experience of sexual aggression, reflected significant reductions in both treatment groups, which were retained at the 13-month followup.

In the RCT by Vaughan and colleagues (1994),[46] applied muscle relaxation (AMR) was compared to eye movement desensitization (EMD) and image habituation training (IHT), a form of exposure therapy. Thirty-six patients with PTSD referred to an outpatient PTSD clinic were randomly assigned to AMR (n = 11), EMD (n = 12), or IHT (n = 13). Participants' trauma histories included violent crime, rape, child abuse, and motor vehicle accident. Schizophrenia and severe personality disorders were exclusions. At baseline, 22 percent reported subclinical levels of Category C (avoidance/numbing) symptoms and thus did not meet full DSM-IIIR criteria for PTSD.

Patients were scheduled to attend four sessions over a 2- to 3-week period. The AMR treatment, adapted from Ost (1987),[53] taught participants to recognize early signs of anxiety and to apply relaxation techniques to manage and quell anxiety. During the treatment sessions, three increasingly brief, relaxation techniques were sequentially introduced: progressive muscle relaxation, release-only relaxation (i.e., passive muscle relaxation), and cue-controlled relaxation, in which self-instruction to "relax" was paired with the state of relaxation. Participants were expected to practice these techniques between sessions, 40 minutes per day. In the EMD condition (now known as eye movement desensitization and reprocessing [EMDR]), saccadic eye movements (induced by asking the patient to track the therapist's hand as it moved rapidly across the visual field) were paired with associative elements of the traumatic memory, including imagery, cognition, affect, and physiological sensations. No between-session work was assigned to participants in the EMD group. Patients in the IHT group were required to listen to continuous-loop, audiotaped descriptions of their trauma and to record cognitions and anxiety levels on a homework sheet for 60 minutes per day. The level of education and training of the therapists was not reported, but all were trained in EMD by Francine Shapiro, the originator of the technique. This study was considered fair quality because of ambiguous reporting of methods (including lack of clarity about the adequacy of randomization, nonblinded assessments, inadequate treatment of missing data, lack of intent-to-treat analyses) and inadequate statistical power.

The primary PTSD-related outcome measure was the PTSD Structured Interview (SI-PTSD), assessed by a blinded rater at baseline, posttreatment (2 to 3 weeks), and 3 months. All three treatment groups were associated with significant improvement ($p < 0.001$) in SI-PTSD scores at the posttreatment and 3-month followup. There were no between-group differences in SI-PTSD scores at the baseline, posttreatment, or 3-month assessments. Adverse effects were not reported.

In a 3-arm, 10-week trial, Watson and colleagues (1997)[47] randomized 90 male Vietnam-era Veterans to 1 of 3 relaxation training conditions: simple relaxation instruction (RI), RI plus deep breathing, or RI plus deep breathing plus thermal biofeedback. All were recruited by a technician at the St. Cloud, Minnesota VA Medical Center; additional details about recruitment procedures were not reported. All met DSM-IIIR criteria for PTSD, per the Posttraumatic Stress Disorder Interview (PTSD-I). Additional details about diagnostic procedures or specific inclusion/exclusion procedures were not provided. The technician, who was trained by a doctoral-level psychologist with 7 years' experience in biofeedback and relaxation therapies, was responsible for recruitment, administration of all study treatments, and all study assessments—and thus was not blinded to treatment group assignment.

All 3 treatment conditions consisted of 10, 30-minute sessions conducted in a quiet, dimly lit laboratory in which participants were seated in a reclining chair and provided 10 minutes to adapt to room temperature before beginning each session. Regardless of treatment group assignment, each participant was attached to a biofeedback apparatus that monitored finger temperature and frontalis muscle tension. Participants randomized to the RI group were instructed to "relax as much as possible" during the sessions. Those in the RI plus deep breathing condition were also given instruction in deep breathing prior to each session and instructed to practice relaxing and deep breathing throughout the 30-minute session. Those in the RI plus deep breathing plus thermal biofeedback condition were additionally told that they would hear a tone, indicating their level of relaxation, and instructed to increase their finger temperature and lower the tone as much as possible by relaxing during the session. Thus, the three treatment arms could be conceptualized as an attention control (RI), relaxation/CAM intervention (RI + deep breathing), and biofeedback/traditional treatment.

Outcomes included PTSD-I total and individual item scores, Mississippi Scale for Combat-Related PTSD (M-PTSD), finger temperature, and frontalis muscle tension. This study was considered poor quality. Key limitations included unclear randomization and allocation concealment; inadequate treatment of incomplete outcome data; nonblinding of subject, provider, and assessor; no intent-to-treat analysis; and no power or sample size calculation/underpowered for comparative analyses. Adverse effects were not reported.

In the completer sample, significant pretreatment versus posttreatment (Week 10) differences were observed for two PTSD symptoms assessed by individual items on the PTSD-I: intrusive memories (p < .01) and exaggerated startle response (p < .05), as well as M-PTSD total scores (p < .05) and middle-finger skin temperature, reported as degrees Fahrenheit p < .05). However, no time-by-treatment group differences were noted. Analysis of outcome data was limited to those who completed at least 9 of the 10 treatment sessions. Those who missed more than one session were replaced by other volunteers; intent-to-treat results were not reported.

To summarize, the findings of three RCTs provided limited support for relaxation interventions for PTSD. However, none of these relatively small studies was adequately powered for comparisons of active treatment groups, and significant design flaws limited interpretability of study findings.

Overall, the findings from six published RCTs that included a mind-body complementary and alternative medicine therapy as an intervention demonstrated the following:

- Meditation techniques were associated with moderate improvements in symptoms and HRQOL compared to usual care only (one fair-quality study) and decreased symptom severity compared to individual psychotherapy (one poor-quality study).
- The clinical effectiveness of a course of acupuncture as a treatment for PTSD was similar to that of group CBT and greater than waitlist control (one good-quality RCT).
- Relaxation training was associated with moderate clinical improvement, but studies were small and favored the active comparator. Because 95 percent confidence intervals were large, an important clinical benefit for active comparators versus relaxation treatment was possible (three poor-quality RCTs).

Unpublished literature

Our search of ClinicalTrials.gov identified 16 RCTs relevant to KQ 1. These studies are summarized in Table 5, organized alphabetically by trial name. We identified eight ongoing trials that are examining the following CAM interventions: acupuncture, emotional freedom techniques, guided imagery/imagery modification, mind-body skills, mindfulness meditation, relaxation, and yoga. In addition, we identified six completed studies for which we could not identify a publication that reported clinical outcomes; they included these interventions: acupuncture, emotional freedom techniques, guided imagery, mindfulness-based stress reduction, and yoga. There was also one trial on yoga with status listed as "unknown." Of the completed studies, two had funding stop dates of April 2009 or earlier, raising the possibility of publication bias for these interventions. The authors of these two studies were contacted, and for one study (Acupuncture for Posttraumatic Stress Among Military Personnel), a manuscript is in development.

Table 5. Ongoing RCTs of mind-body interventions (KQ 1)

Study title	VA/DoD population?	Intervention	Comparator	Sponsor and clinicaltrials.gov ID	Funding start and stop date	Status
A Controlled Breathing Course for Social & Emotional Health for Vietnam Veterans with Chronic PTSD-RCT[a]	Y	Yoga breathing technique; single group assignment	Not clearly specified	The University of Queensland NCT00256477	Mar 2005–Oct 2005	Completed[b]
Acupuncture for the Treatment of Posttraumatic Stress Among Military Personnel[a]	Y	Acupuncture	Waitlist	Henry M. Jackson Foundation NCT00320138	Mar 2006–Oct 2007	Completed
Effectiveness of Three Different Psychotherapies for Chronic Post-Traumatic Stress Disorder	N	Interpersonal psychotherapy	1. Prolonged exposure 2. Relaxation	NIMH NCT00739765	Apr 2008–Mar 2013	Recruiting
Effect of EFT on Psychological States in a Veterans Population[a]	Y	Emotional Freedom Techniques	Standard care	Soul Medicine Institute NCT0074341	Dec 2008– May 2010	Completed
Efficacy of Yoga for Treatment-Resistant Posttraumatic Stress Disorder	N	Yoga	Women's health education	Justice Resource Institute NCT00839813	Nov 2008–May 2011	Recruiting
Evaluation of a MCYI as Adjunct of Psychiatric Treatment for Vietnam Veterans With PTSD-RCT[a]	Y	Yoga	Usual care	The University of Queensland NCT00256464	Jun 2007–Jan 2008	Unknown
Evaluation of Telehealth Interventions for Post-Trauma Stress[a]	Y	Mindfulness Telehealth Intervention	Self	Samueli Institute for Information Biology NCT00350584	Feb 2007–Apr 2008	Completed
Examining the Effect of Acupuncture on Sleep Difficulties Related to Post Traumatic Stress Disorder	Y	Acupuncture	1. Sham acupuncture 2. No intervention	Department of Veterans Affairs NCT00866517	Oct 2009–Sep 2011	Recruiting
Guided Imagery for Military Sexual Trauma-Related Posttraumatic Stress Disorder (PTSD)[a]	Y	Guided imagery	Music	Duke University NCT00635635	Oct 2007–Mar 2010	Completed

Efficacy of Complementary and Alternative Medicine Therapies for Posttraumatic Stress Disorder

Study title	VA/DoD population?	Intervention	Comparator	Sponsor and clinicaltrials.gov ID	Funding start and stop date	Status
Mechanistic Pathways of Mindfulness Meditation in Post-Traumatic Stress Disorder	Y	1. Slow breathing 2. Meditation 3. Meditation + slow breathing	Sitting quietly	Oregon Health and Science University NCT00778960	Jan 2009–Sep 2013	Recruiting
Mind-Body Skills Groups for the Treatment of War Zone Stress in Military and Veteran Populations	Y	Mind-body skills	Standard treatment	The Center for Mind-Body Medicine NCT01093053	Sep 2010–Aug 2012	Recruiting
Mindfulness Based Stress Reduction for Posttraumatic Stress Disorder: A Pilot Study[a]	Y	Mindfulness-based stress reduction	Usual care	Seattle Institute for Biomedical and Clinical Research NCT00880152	Sep 2008–Dec 2009	Completed
Neural Correlates of PTSD Prevention With Mindfulness Based Stress Reduction (MBSR) in Iraqi Veterans[a]	Y	Mindfulness-based stress reduction	Supportive therapy	Department of Veterans Affairs NCT01058031	Jan 2007–Nov 2010	Completed
Pilot of Acupuncture to Improve Quality of life in Veterans with Traumatic Brain Injury (TBI) and Post-Traumatic Stress Disorder (PTSD)	Y	Acupuncture	Standard care	Department of Veterans Affairs NCT01060553	Jul 2010–Jun 2011	Recruiting
Psychological Symptom Change in Veterans After Six Sessions of EFT (Emotional Freedom Technique)	Y	Emotional Freedom Technique	Waitlist	Soul Medicine Institute NCT01117545	May 2010–Jun 2013	Recruiting
Study on the Psychotherapeutic Treatment for the Feeling of Being Contaminated After Childhood Sexual Abuse	N	Imagery modification	Waitlist	Goethe University NCT00976859	Sep 2009–Dec 2011	Recruiting

[a]No publication found.

[b]Author contacted, no results published in peer-reviewed journal as of May 2011.

Abbreviations: NCCAM = National Center for Complementary and Alternative Medicine, NIMH = National Institute of Mental Health, PTSD = posttraumatic stress disorder, RCT = randomized controlled trial

KEY QUESTION 2: In adults with PTSD, are manipulative and body-based complementary and alternative medicine therapies (e.g., spinal manipulation, massage) more efficacious than control for PTSD symptoms and health-related quality of life?

Published literature

We identified one poor-quality RCT by Price (2006)[48,49] of body-oriented therapy in eight adult female subjects with histories of childhood sexual trauma (Table 6).

Table 6. Characteristics of manipulative and body-based interventions (KQ 2)

Study	Population	Design details	Intervention	Comparator	Outcomes[a]
Price, 2006[48,49]	N = 8 Trauma: rape, childhood physical/ sexual abuse Mean age (SD): 38 (NR) Women: 8 (100%) Veterans: none	PTSD diagnosis: Severity of PTSD by PCL Key exclusions: Substance abuse, currently involved in a violent relationship, Not currently in active psychotherapy, Not able to pay 50% of the cost for massage Recruitment: clinical referral	8 weekly 60-minute sessions of body-oriented therapy (massage) + body awareness education and body-mind integration	Waitlist	Remission: Score below clinical cut-off— intervention group, 2 of 4 vs. waitlist group, 1 of 4 Response: symptom improvement, intervention group, p < .01 HRQOL = NR AE = NR Followup duration: 9 weeks (end of treatment)

[a]If comparator, outcomes given for intervention versus comparator.

Abbreviations: AE = adverse effect, NR = not reported, HRQOL = health-related quality of life, PCL = PTSD Checklist

Although formal PTSD diagnosis was not a study inclusion criterion, six of the eight women screened positive for PTSD at study inception, as indicated by baseline administration of the Crime-Related Post Traumatic Stress Disorder Scale (CR-PTSD)—the primary outcome variable. Participants were recruited through clinician referral, free advertisements on women's groups' Web sites, and emails to select graduate students; no VA or DoD settings were included. To be included, women had to be in active psychotherapy; be willing to stop any current bodywork one month prior to entering the study; and agree to pay 50 percent of the cost for the study-related bodywork sessions. Exclusion criteria were current substance abuse, involvement in a violent relationship, or psychiatric hospitalization within the last year. There was no requirement to maintain stable dosages of psychotropic medications. Four subjects were randomly allocated to eight, 1-hour sessions of Swedish-type massage, body awareness education, and "body-mind integration" (i.e., exploration of links between internal experiences and physiological sensations). The other four subjects were allocated to a waitlist control. The primary outcome measure, assessed at 9 weeks, was the CR-PTSD.

Pretreatment and posttreatment (Week 9) changes in scores were presented graphically, but axis labels were unclear, which hampered interpretation. Study limitations included incomplete descriptions of study participants, small sample size, and the potential for differing cointerventions across groups. In addition, the principal investigator collected and analyzed all data, and was not blinded to treatment condition. Although not explicitly stated, it appeared that the principal investigator also was the sole interventionist; her level of experience providing bodywork was not stated. This limitation introduces potential bias and confounds treatment and therapist effects. As is common for a small preliminary study, treatment adherence and fidelity were not assessed.

The sample was relatively homogeneous: 89 percent were white; 71 percent reported incomes equal to or greater than $25,000; and all had at least a bachelor-level education. Sexual orientation was fairly varied—nearly half reported homosexual or bisexual orientations. All subjects had been in psychotherapy at least 1 year (range 1 to 20), and five of eight women were taking psychotropic medications. By Week 9, clinical remission (per recommended screening cutoffs on the CR-PTSD) had occurred in two of four women in the intervention group and one of four women in the waitlist control group. Pretreatment and posttreatment within-group comparisons showed significant improvements for the intervention group but not for the control group on the CR-PTSD; between-group comparisons were not significant.

In summary, the findings from one small, poor-quality RCT in a relatively homogeneous sample provided modest support for the application of body-oriented therapy as an adjunctive treatment for women survivors of childhood sexual assault. We found no RCTs of manipulative or body-based CAM interventions in men, military or Veteran samples, or individuals with PTSD related to more recent traumatic stressors (versus childhood abuse). We were unable to identify published RCTs of other manipulative or body-based CAM interventions, such as chiropractic medicine and naturopathy, or of alternative applications and forms of massage therapy.

Unpublished literature

Our search of ClinicalTrials.gov did not identify any RCTs relevant to KQ 2.

KEY QUESTION 3: In adults with PTSD, are complementary and alternative medicine therapies that are movement-based or involve energy therapies more efficacious than control for PTSD and health-related quality of life?

Our literature search identified no published RCTs of movement-based or energy therapies for PTSD.

Unpublished literature

Our search of ClinicalTrials.gov did not identify any RCTs relevant to KQ 3.

KEY QUESTION 4: For treatments evaluated in KQs 1–3 that lack RCTs, is there evidence from other study designs that suggests the potential for treatment efficacy?

Published literature

We identified two nonrandomized, prospective studies (Table 7) that assessed clinical outcomes over time among patients with PTSD who received a CAM intervention as defined in the Methods section.

Table 7. Characteristics of nonrandomized CAM treatment studies (KQ 4)

Study	Population	Design details	Intervention	Comparator	Outcomes
Abramowitz and Lichtenberg, 2010[50]	Israeli combat Veterans with PTSD by DSM-IV. Mean age: 41.2 (12.2) Women: 0% Veterans: 100%	Prospective cohort (N = 36) Outcomes: 1. Immediately posttreatment (6 weeks) 2. 6 months 3. 1 year	Hypnotherapeutic olfactory conditioning Six 1.5-hour sessions over 6 weeks	NA	Remission: NR Response: IES-R; improvement was significant at the 6-week posttreatment assessment and remained improved at 6 and 12 months
Hossack and Bentall, 1996[51]	Male volunteers who met DSM-III-R criteria for PTSD Mean age: 34.8 (10.26) Women: 0% Veterans: 0%	Multiple baseline design across subjects (N = 5) Outcome: Subjects 1 and 2 received intervention at 3 weeks from baseline; subject 3 received intervention at 6 weeks from baseline; subjects 4 and 5 received intervention at 9 weeks from baseline	4 therapy sessions including Relaxation: Jacobson's method and guided imagery Two sessions Visual kinesthetic dissociation Two sessions	Baseline	Response: 3 patients reported decrease in intrusive imagery, 1 reported "less clear cut improvement," and 1 showed "no improvement"

Abbreviations: DSM = Diagnostic and Statistical Manual of Mental Disorders, IES-R = Impact of Events Scale-Revised, NA = not applicable, NR = not reported, PTSD = posttraumatic stress disorder

A prospective cohort study by Abramowitz and Lichtenberg (2010)[50] involved 36 Israeli veterans with combat-related PTSD and treatment-resistant, olfactory-induced flashbacks. DSM-IV diagnostic criteria were determined by semistructured, clinical interview. Participants underwent a form of brief hypnotherapy that entailed six, 90-minute, weekly hypnotherapeutic olfactory conditioning sessions in addition to standard CBT and stress management strategies (including imaginal exposure to the traumatic event). The core components of the intervention included:

- Session 1: repeated pairing of pleasant memories with a pleasant-smelling essential oil (i.e., classical conditioning)
- Session 2: hypnotic induction, imaginal reexperiencing of functioning well under stress,

paired with hypnotic suggestion that the participant can manage PTSD-related intrusive memories and flashbacks

- Session 3: use of guided imagery, hypnosis, and suggestion around themes of mastery, control, and safety, paired with the pleasant scent identified in the initial session
- Sessions 4 and 5: repeated imaginal exposure to traumatic memories under hypnosis, paired with the pleasant scent
- Session 6: review of treatment gains, new skills, and plans to maintain and use new skills, particularly when triggered by olfactory stimuli

Compared to baseline, the Impact of Events Scale-Revised (IES-R) scores were significantly improved at 6 weeks, 6 months, and 12 months. The investigators also reported significant decreases at 12 months, relative to baseline, in dosage and use of SSRIs, benzodiazepine, and neuroleptic medications.

The multiple baseline case series by Hossack and Bentall (1996)[51] examined a visual-kinesthetic dissociation intervention in five male U.K. residents who reported severe intrusive imagery and met DSM-IIIR criteria for PTSD. Study diagnoses were determined by forensic psychiatrists and confirmed by brief clinical interview by the lead author. Participants' trauma histories included surviving an industrial helicopter crash (n = 1) and witnessing a crowd surge at a football stadium that resulted in 95 deaths (n = 4). In addition to the five participants who completed treatment, a sixth participant enrolled but dropped out during the baseline phase and was not included in study analyses. The Impact of Events Scale (IES), which assesses Cluster B ("reexperiencing") and Cluster C ("avoidance and numbing") symptoms, was the primary measure of PTSD severity. Participants also completed daily diaries of duration, clarity, and related distress. The four-session intervention was administered in two phases:

- Relaxation: In the first two individual sessions, participants were taught to apply progressive muscle relaxation and guided imagery techniques to promote relaxation. Instruction in guided imagery emphasized incorporation of multiple sensory modalities (visual, kinesthetic, auditory, olfactory, and gustatory) in preparation for the next treatment phase.
- Visual-kinesthetic dissociation: In the final two sessions, participants were taught to apply relaxation skills and multisensory imagery techniques to imagine themselves at the cinema and to switch vantage points between being within a film of their trauma (first person), watching the film (second person), and watching themselves watch the film (third person). Using a manualized protocol, participants were then taught to manipulate the color and speed of the film and to run it backward and forward while repeatedly rotating their experience of the image from the first-, second-, and third-person perspectives.

In addition to daily diaries of intrusive events, assessments were conducted at regular intervals across the 17 weeks in which this multiple baseline design study was conducted, as well as 3-month followup (29-week assessment). No descriptive or inferential statistical analyses were conducted. However, visual plots of each participant's symptom change over time were presented and discussed. The authors report "substantial" reductions in IES scores for four of the five participants (although two showed evidence of some posttreatment increase in avoidance).

Daily diary results indicated that four participants reported sizable decreases in the experience of intrusive imagery (maintained at 3-month followup), whereas one experienced a modest increase. The authors noted that daily diary results suggested important (albeit preliminary) differences in how participants responded to the different treatment components: for one participant, relaxation seemed the most potent; for another, visual-kinesthetic dissociation had the greatest impact; and two others seemed to respond to both interventions.

In summary, the two published, nonrandomized studies identified by our systematic search provided little evidence of broad potential efficacy in PTSD for any of the CAM interventions of interest. One study[50] presented initial pilot findings of a multimodal intervention that included both CAM (hypnotherapy, guided imagery) and imaginal exposure techniques. Although initial findings are promising, the study appears most applicable to the subgroup of combat Veterans who are particularly sensitive to olfactory triggers. Because the study sample was limited to men, it provided no additional information about the potential efficacy of CAM modalities in women. Likewise, a second study in five males provided limited initial information about the feasibility and potential utility of brief CAM intervention that included instruction in relaxation skills and imagery techniques including imaginal exposure.

In addition to these studies, one additional nonrandomized study,[54] which was published after we conducted our literature search, was identified during the peer review process. In a study by Rosenthal and colleagues (2011), five OEF/OIF Veterans who met DSM-IV diagnostic criteria for combat-related PTSD were instructed in transcendental meditation (TM) by a certified instructor and asked to practice the technique for 20 minutes, twice daily, during the 12-week study period. Clinician support was provided through the study duration via biweekly, face-to-face meetings, as well as telephone, email, and text message contacts. At 8-week followup, patients showed improvements in the clinician-rated PTSD symptom severity (CAPS: M change score = 31.4, p = 0.02), self-reported PTSD symptom severity (PCL: M change score = 24.00, p < .02), and self-reported quality of life (Q-LES-Q-SF: M change score = -13.00, p < 0.01). The results of this small, uncontrolled study provide additional preliminary support for applications of meditation in Veterans with PTSD.[54]

Unpublished literature

Our search of ClinicalTrials.gov identified two non-RCTs relevant to KQ 4. These studies are summarized in Table 8, organized alphabetically by trial name. Both trials examined yoga. One is still recruiting, but the other is completed with a funding stop date of April 2009 or earlier, raising the possibility of publication bias for this intervention.

Table 8. Nonrandomized studies (KQ 4)

Study Title	VA/DOD population?	Intervention	Comparator	Sponsor and clinicaltrials.gov ID	Funding start and stop date	Status
Evaluation of a Yoga Intervention for Post-Traumatic Stress Disorder	Y	Yoga	None	Brigham and Women's Hospital NCT00962403	Aug 2009–Dec 2010	Recruiting
Yoga as a Therapy for Traumatic Experience[a]	Y	Yoga	None	Samueli Institute for Information Biology NCT00269490	Dec 2005–Aug 2007	Completed

[a]No publication found

SUMMARY AND DISCUSSION

This evidence synthesis was requested by VA Research and Development to review and summarize the empirical evidence for applications of common CAM therapies to the treatment of PTSD. Four KQs were identified to examine the efficacy of mind-body therapies (KQ 1), manipulative and body-based therapies (KQ 2), movement-based therapies (KQ 3), and relevant evidence derived from nonrandomized trials of CAM interventions for PTSD (KQ 4).

Our systematic literature search yielded six RCTs relevant to KQ 1, one relevant to KQ 2, and none to KQ 3. For KQ 4, which enabled us to expand our search beyond RCTs to include nonrandomized trials, two additional studies were identified. Most studies reviewed appeared to be preliminary investigations and were underpowered, limited by significant design flaws, and often provided inadequate descriptions of the intervention to permit replication. For each KQ, the evidence reviewed was limited. Indeed, perhaps our most striking finding overall was the relative dearth of available evidence on CAM applications for PTSD, despite clear consumer interest and widespread use of these treatments.

SUMMARY OF EVIDENCE BY KEY QUESTION

For each KQ, we summarize the strength of evidence (SOE) and magnitude of treatment effects in Table 9. Interventions are compared to control or usual care and to active treatments separately. When the strength of evidence was rated insufficient, we did not calculate a treatment effect.

Table 9. Summary of the strength of evidence for KQs 1–3

Number of studies (subjects)	Domains pertaining to strength of evidence				Magnitude of effect[a] and SOE
	Risk of bias: design/quality	Consistency	Directness	Precision	PTSD symptoms: Effect estimate (95% CI)
KQ 1: Meditation vs. usual care					**Low SOE**
1 (29)	RCT/Fair	Not applicable	Direct	Imprecise	SMD: -0.32 (-1.46 to 0.05), self-report PCL; -0.70 (-1.06 to 0.41), interviewer-based CAPS
KQ 1: Meditation vs. active treatment					**Insufficient SOE**
1 (26)	RCT/Poor	Not applicable	Direct	Imprecise	Not estimated
KQ 1: Acupuncture vs. control					**Moderate SOE**
1 (84)	RCT/Good	Not applicable	Direct	Imprecise	SMD: -0.92 (-1.51 to -0.32), self-report PSS-SR
KQ 1: Acupuncture vs. group CBT					**Low SOE**
1 (84)	RCT/Good	Not applicable	Direct	Imprecise	SMD: -0.35 (-0.91 to 0.22), self-report PSS-SR
KQ 1: Relaxation vs. control					**Insufficient SOE**
1 (90)	RCT/Poor	Not applicable	Direct	Imprecise	Not estimated

Number of studies (subjects)	Domains pertaining to strength of evidence				Magnitude of effect[a] and SOE
KQ 1: Relaxation vs. other active treatment					**Insufficient SOE**
2 (56)	RCT/Fair to Poor	Consistent	Direct	Imprecise	Low[b] SMD: 0.41 (-0.42 to 1.24), interviewer based SI-PTSD SMD: 0.79 (-0.13 to 1.71), interviewer based SS-PTSD
KQ 2: Massage vs. control					**Insufficient SOE**
1 (8)	RCT/Fair	Not applicable	Direct	Imprecise	Not estimated
KQ 3: Movement-based and energy therapies vs. control					**Insufficient SOE**
None	NA	NA	NA	NA	NA

[a]A negative SMD indicates a greater effect for the CAM therapy.

[b]SMDs were are reported separately for the two studies because a summary estimate was not indicated.

Abbreviations: CI = confidence interval, OR = odds ratio, NA = not applicable, RCT = randomized controlled trial, SMD = standardized mean difference, SOE = strength of evidence

Considered in sum, the highest quality evidence exists for acupuncture. However, strong conclusions cannot reliably be drawn on the basis of a single RCT; replication of findings is required. In addition, the active comparator in this study was group CBT, which is generally considered to be less potent than individual CBT therapies.[55] The greatest breadth of evidence exists for relaxation interventions—we identified three RCTs that examined forms of breathing and muscle relaxation. In each case, the trials were preliminary and design flaws limited interpretation of study findings, which were positive overall. Further conclusions cannot be made in the absence of well-designed investigations of these modalities.

The evidence base for meditation therapies is similarly limited by a paucity of well-designed trials, although early evidence is promising. In addition to a lack of scientific rigor and the need to replicate preliminary findings, the current literature is limited to concentrative meditative techniques. No RCTs of other common mind-body interventions, including mindfulness meditation and yoga, were identified in our review of the published, peer-reviewed literature. However, we identified 16 ongoing and/or unpublished studies registered with ClinicalTrials.gov, suggesting that this is a growing area of research. Approximately half of these trials are ongoing, and the majority are recruiting active military and/or Veteran samples. Thus, a significantly larger and broader evidence base may be anticipated within the next several years.

For manipulative and body-based CAM therapies, the evidence base is extremely limited, and for movement-based and energy therapies, we identified no RCTs, published or in progress. Thus, the current and developing evidence bases for these therapies are likely to remain insufficient for clinical or policy recommendations in the near future.

More broadly, the limitations of the current evidence preclude conclusions about specific interventions, populations, formats, settings, appropriate treatment length or "dosing," or other refinements to the development of these approaches. We found little evidence addressing adverse effects, and retention rates, when reported, were comparable to current evidence-based treatments.

LIMITATIONS

Several limitations of the current review merit mention. First, we limited our literature search to clinical trials published in peer-reviewed, English-language journals. We also searched ClinicalTrials.gov for ongoing and unpublished trials, which served as a proxy "snapshot" of additional evidence that may be anticipated in the near future. However, our search did not extend to the "gray literature," and thus excluded technical reports, white papers, and other evidence streams and formats that would not have been identified through standard database searches. In addition, we limited our literature search to CAM trials conducted in PTSD samples. Thus, the current review did not consider evidence of CAM applications in other anxiety disorders, major depression, or sleep disorders, for which there is symptom overlap and frequent comorbidity with PTSD. For example, in their review of CAM and self-help treatments for all anxiety disorders (generalized anxiety disorder was most frequently described), Jorm and colleagues[56] found evidence from at least one well-designed RCT in support of acupuncture, aromatherapy, massage, dance and movement, meditation, relaxation training, and yoga. Other recent evidence reviews and meta-analyses have examined applications of massage in depression;[57] energy therapies for health and mental health conditions;[58] mindfulness-based stress reduction for anxiety, depression, pain, and chronic medical conditions;[59-61] meditation therapy in anxiety disorders;[62] and vipassana (mindfulness) meditation in a broad range of presentations.[63] Evidence of effectiveness in closely related mental illnesses could provide indirect evidence of effectiveness for PTSD.

The current review also did not include applications of CAM treatments in nonclinical populations or noninterventional designs. Because relaxation training has been employed as a placebo control condition in PTSD treatment trials, our inclusion criteria specified that relaxation interventions be presented as active treatment and that the key components be described in sufficient detail. These criteria led to the exclusion of five RCTs of relaxation interventions for PTSD, which otherwise would have met criteria for inclusion in the current review. Of these, two were excluded because relaxation was a control rather than an active comparator,[37,38] and three were excluded due to lack of detail about the relaxation condition, such that we could not confidently categorize the interventions as CAM.[39-41] It merits mention that in these studies, relaxation showed modest effects and performed less favorability than active comparators. Thus, a wider set of inclusion criteria for the current review may have yielded a larger evidence base, and tempered enthusiasm for applications of relaxation-based monotherapies for PTSD. Likewise, we did not examine, or attempt to examine, issues of symptom overlap or comorbidity of PTSD and traumatic brain injury or other unique presentations that may be anticipated among OEF/OIF Veterans. In addition, the scope of our literature search excluded natural products (e.g., nutritional supplements), as was our charge. Finally, our review did not examine third-wave psychotherapies (e.g., mindfulness-based cognitive therapy, dialectical behavior therapy, and acceptance and commitment therapy) and related approaches. Despite some conceptual overlap with CAM and incorporation of CAM techniques such as meditation, these approaches are theoretically grounded in cognitive behavioral theory. They are understood to be extensions of mainstream approaches—and thus are distinct from CAM. Although outside of the scope of the current review, consideration of these strategies may inform broader understanding of the utility of CAM approaches for PTSD. It also merits mention that numerous forms and practices of mindfulness practice exist, such as seated meditation, movement-based practices, and even the occasional mindful enjoyment of a single raisin. The field may be best served at this stage of treatment development by considering a range of different approaches to cultivating mindfulness skills.

In addition to the above limitations, there are important strengths of our methodological approach as well. First, limiting our review to evidence gleaned from published, peer-reviewed trials allowed us to focus on quality over quantity when examining this relatively undeveloped body of research. Although many CAM approaches have been in practice for thousands of years, the application of rigorous methods to standardize and evaluate the efficacy of these treatments is a relatively new development in the field of interventional PTSD research. In addition, our evidence synthesis was guided by a carefully designed standardized protocol, including a systematic search of research databases and relevant bibliographies, double data abstraction, and use of AHRQ criteria to assess the quality of identified studies. Our multidisciplinary team included expertise in internal medicine, clinical psychology, epidemiology, acupuncture research, and integrative medicine. In sum, this was a highly structured and systematic review of the extant evidence.

RECOMMENDATIONS FOR FUTURE RESEARCH

The limitations of the current evidence preclude our ability to draw strong conclusions to inform clinical practice or public policy regarding optimal use of CAM therapies for PTSD, yet the limitations in the available evidence point to numerous opportunities for future research. Questions remain about the efficacy, effectiveness, safety, cost-effectiveness, comparative effectiveness, mechanisms of actions, dosing, indications and contraindications, and differential response among subgroup populations. There are also unanswered questions about patient and provider preferences and expectations, optimal outcome, adherence and fidelity measures, and resource utilization patterns.

One of the most pertinent questions regarding CAM therapies for PTSD is, What effects might one expect of a given intervention relative to no intervention? This clinically relevant question is best addressed by a randomized clinical trial with a no-treatment (waitlist) comparator. This trial design controls for many threats to internal validity and is particularly appropriate when there are no or few controlled trials. However, study designs that withhold or delay treatment to those with PTSD may not be institutionally feasible or ethically defensible.[64] In their thoughtful discussion of the methodological challenges inherent in this area of research, Devilly and McFarlane (2009)[65] question the value and appropriateness of waitlist and placebo-controlled PTSD intervention trials given potential risks (e.g., greater chronicity, comorbidities, suicidality, functional impairments, and financial burden) that may be incurred when available evidence-based treatments are withheld or delayed. As an alternative to the standard RCT design, the authors demonstrate a means of deriving statistical estimates of waitlist control and placebo treatment effect sizes from existing data and applying these estimates to interpret the effects of future treatment innovations. Although this statistical approach has not been used widely, such strategies merit consideration as an alternative to the use of nonactive controls.

Another pertinent question is, To what extent might placebo, or nonspecific effects account for observed clinical outcomes? This question can be hard to answer for CAM therapies, for which it may be difficult to design a sham procedure that is both truly inert and that appears sufficiently similar to the active intervention to isolate the specific effect of the intervention. The fields of surgical and psychotherapy research have long grappled with similar issues. Strong recommendations and methodological guidelines now exist to guide these efforts. [66,67] Of the many CAM therapies with potential to serve as a therapeutic option in the treatment of PTSD, acupuncture is arguably the one with the most plausible placebo control. For example, it is possible, in the context of a clinical trial, to administer sham acupuncture such that research subjects are unable to determine with certainty whether they are receiving the true or sham treatment. The current standard in acupuncture research is to compare an active acupuncture intervention to both a sham acupuncture intervention and a no-acupuncture control. This three-arm RCT design makes it possible to simultaneously assess the efficacy or effectiveness and safety of a course of acupuncture while also partially addressing the extent to which nonspecific effects may contribute to observed outcomes.

Although more costly and challenging to conduct, comparative effectiveness designs also may be indicated to give patients and clinicians the most direct evidence about competing treatment options. These trials may be most appropriate and informative after additional preliminary work has fostered a stronger evidence base for CAM treatments of interest. Finally, practical clinical trials, which combine aspects of efficacy and effectiveness designs, merit consideration as a potentially more efficient and actionable alternative to traditional explanatory trials.[68]

Ultimately, the choice of which research strategy to employ should be determined by the key questions and the plausibility and estimates of benefit based on prior research.[66,69-71] For example, explanatory trials are best suited to address the question, Can this intervention work? and pragmatic trials to address the question, Does this intervention work?[69] For most CAM treatments, the basic question of "Can it work?" for PTSD has not been answered. Observational studies can provide good evidence about the feasibility of interventions and adverse effects that require large studies or long followup durations to detect. Smeeding and colleagues (2010)[72] conducted a longitudinal evaluation of the effectiveness of an integrative health clinic and program within the Veterans Affairs Health Care System (VAHCS) for PTSD, chronic pain, stress-related depression, and anxiety. Observational studies of this kind can provide a rich source of information about the feasibility and acceptability of CAM treatments delivered within a VA setting. In addition, high-quality observational studies that show very large treatment effects can provide good evidence of treatment effect. For example, we do not need an RCT to prove the benefits of a good parachute when stepping out of an airplane at altitude. However, our review did not identify observational studies showing very large treatment effects for any of the CAM treatments evaluated. Thus, randomized, placebo (or sham intervention) controlled trials— the gold standard for evaluating intervention effects—will be the most logical design for the majority of studies planned to evaluate CAM interventions. Small exploratory trials would be a logical next step for the CAM interventions that lack any studies of treatment effect.[67]

Whether evaluated in RCTs or observational studies, evaluating CAM therapies is challenging.[73,74] A complete description of the challenges is beyond the scope of this report, but issues of blinding patients and treating clinicians to the intervention assignment, accounting for the learning curve of procedural-based interventions, identifying the appropriate comparator, procedures to minimize attrition, and monitoring fidelity to the planned intervention are all key challenges. In addition, research on PTSD has important challenges, including the variety of traumas (e.g., combat, rape), the time since trauma, and the presence of medical or psychiatric comorbidity, all of which may impact treatment response. In addition to these more general challenges, we observed important variability in the completeness and consistency of PTSD outcome reporting. The evidence base for CAM treatments, and PTSD more generally, would be strengthened by a more uniform approach to outcome assessment. For our review, we prioritized PTSD symptom response, HRQOL, and adverse effects as the most important outcomes. Secondary outcomes included patient satisfaction, treatment adherence, and functional status. This prioritization of outcomes should be confirmed with stakeholders and then assessed more consistently across studies. To this end, the PROMIS initiative, an AHRQ-funded effort to develop a common battery of measures for many different conditions, may be a useful resource. Another important limitation of the current evidence base was the descriptions of treatment interventions, which were usually inadequate to permit replication. Glasziou and colleagues[75] have recently proposed standards for intervention reporting to include sufficient detail to guide replication, including descriptions of the interventionists, the content of the intervention, the treatment setting, how and when the intervention was delivered, and the degree of flexibility permissible. Finally, health services research in the VA could be facilitated by developing procedure codes to capture CAM approaches used in the VA.

CONCLUSIONS

Our systematic review identified seven RCTs and two nonrandomized studies of CAM interventions for PTSD. Our review of relevant studies registered with ClinicalTrials.gov further suggests that this modest empirical foundation is growing. The term CAM encompasses a broad range of treatments—not all of which may hold the same level of promise as applications for PTSD. The current absence of a strong signal pointing to any one CAM approach over others argues for investment in a set of adequately powered trials to evaluate the most promising therapies, rather than a single large trial for any one treatment. Given the current state of evidence, a two-pronged approach may be most appropriate at this stage to move the field forward. That is, a series of adequately powered RCTs may be indicated for select CAM interventions for which there is clear and strong preliminary signal, either based on good-quality, early empirical evidence (e.g., acupuncture), a sound theoretical rationale for efficacy in the absence of strong pilot findings (e.g., meditation), and/or promising data gleaned from the bench sciences (e.g., compelling animal models). For other CAM modalities for which the science and theory are even less well developed, such as energy therapies, more prudence is indicated, suggesting the utility of exploratory pilot studies as the appropriate next step. In addition, the efficiency and ultimate yield of future efforts may be further optimized by consensus agreement about, and concerted efforts to address, limitations identified in the current literature. Broadly, these limitations concern issues of appropriate design, outcome, and replication strategies. There is an opportunity for strategic, well-designed studies to address the substantial gaps in evidence identified in this review.

REFERENCES

1. Kessler RC, Berglund P, Demler O, et al. Lifetime prevalence and age-of-onset distributions of DSM-IV disorders in the National Comorbidity Survey Replication. *Arch Gen Psychiatry*. 2005;62(6):593-602.

2. Amaya-Jackson L, Davidson JR, Hughes DC, et al. Functional impairment and utilization of services associated with posttraumatic stress in the community. *J Trauma Stress*. 1999;12(4):709-24.

3. Calhoun PS, Bosworth HB, Grambow SC, et al. Medical service utilization by veterans seeking help for posttraumatic stress disorder. *Am J Psychiatry*. 2002;159(12):2081-6.

4. Helzer JE, Robins LN, McEvoy L. Post-traumatic stress disorder in the general population. Findings of the epidemiologic catchment area survey. *N Engl J Med*. 1987;317(26):1630-4.

5. Hoge CW, Terhakopian A, Castro CA, et al. Association of posttraumatic stress disorder with somatic symptoms, health care visits, and absenteeism among Iraq war veterans. *Am J Psychiatry*. 2007;164(1):150-3.

6. Jakupcak M, Cook J, Imel Z, et al. Posttraumatic stress disorder as a risk factor for suicidal ideation in Iraq and Afghanistan War veterans. *J Trauma Stress*. 2009;22(4):303-6.

7. Prigerson HG, Maciejewski PK, Rosenheck RA. Population attributable fractions of psychiatric disorders and behavioral outcomes associated with combat exposure among US men. *Am J Public Health*. 2002;92(1):59-63.

8. Thomas JL, Wilk JE, Riviere LA, et al. Prevalence of mental health problems and functional impairment among active component and National Guard soldiers 3 and 12 months following combat in Iraq. *Arch Gen Psychiatry*. 2010;67(6):614-23.

9. Weisberg RB, Bruce SE, Machan JT, et al. Nonpsychiatric illness among primary care patients with trauma histories and posttraumatic stress disorder. *Psychiatr Serv*. 2002;53(7):848-54.

10. Hosek JR, United States. Dept. of Defense. Office of the Secretary of Defense., National Defense Research Institute (U.S.). *How is deployment to Iraq and Afghanistan affecting U.S. service members and their families? An overview of early RAND research on the topic*. Santa Monica, CA: RAND Corporation; 2011.

11. Seal KH, Metzler TJ, Gima KS, et al. Trends and risk factors for mental health diagnoses among Iraq and Afghanistan veterans using Department of Veterans Affairs health care, 2002-2008. *Am J Public Health*. 2009;99(9):1651-8.

12. Rosenheck RA, Fontana AF. Recent Trends In VA Treatment Of Post-Traumatic Stress Disorder And Other Mental. *Health Aff (Millwood)*. 2007:1720-1727.

13. Kessler RC, Davis RB, Foster DF, et al. Long-term trends in the use of complementary and alternative medical therapies in the United States. *Ann Intern Med*. 2001;135(4):262-8.

14. Barnes PM, Bloom B, Nahin RL. Complementary and alternative medicine use among adults and children: United States, 2007. National health statistics reports; no 12. Hyattsville, MD: National Center for Health Statistics. 2008. Available at: http://nccam.nih.gov/news/2008/nhsr12.pdf. Accessed May 31, 2011.

15. Unutzer J, Klap R, Sturm R, et al. Mental disorders and the use of alternative medicine: results from a national survey. *Am J Psychiatry*. 2000;157(11):1851-7.

16. The Management of Post-Traumatic Stress Working Group. VA/DoD Clinical Practice Guideline for Management of Post-Traumatic Stress. 2010.

17. Bisson J, Andrew M. Psychological treatment of post-traumatic stress disorder (PTSD). *Cochrane Database Syst Rev*. 2007(3):CD003388.

18. Foa EB, International Society for Traumatic Stress Studies. *Effective treatments for PTSD: practice guidelines from the International Society for Traumatic Stress Studies*. 2nd ed New York: Guilford Press; 2009.

19. Institute of Medicine (IOM). *Treatment of posttraumatic stress disorder: An assessment of the evidence.* Washington, DC: The National Academies Press; 2008.

20. Bradley R, Greene J, Russ E, et al. A multidimensional meta-analysis of psychotherapy for PTSD. *Am J Psychiatry*. 2005;162(2):214-27.

21. Stein DJ, Ipser JC, Seedat S. Pharmacotherapy for post traumatic stress disorder (PTSD). *Cochrane Database Syst Rev*. 2006(1):CD002795.

22. Zohar J, Amital D, Miodownik C, et al. Double-blind placebo-controlled pilot study of sertraline in military veterans with posttraumatic stress disorder. *J Clin Psychopharmacol*. 2002;22(2):190-5.

23. Davidson J, Baldwin D, Stein DJ, et al. Treatment of posttraumatic stress disorder with venlafaxine extended release: A 6-month randomized controlled trial. *Arch Gen Psychiatry*. 2006;63(10):1158-1165.

24. Hoge CW, Castro CA, Messer SC, et al. Combat duty in Iraq and Afghanistan, mental health problems, and barriers to care. *N Engl J Med*. 2004;351(1):13-22.

25. Feeny NC, Zoellner LA, Mavissakalian MR, et al. What would you choose? Sertraline or prolonged exposure in community and PTSD treatment seeking women. *Depress Anxiety*. 2009;26(8):724-31.

26. Anderson IM. Selective serotonin reuptake inhibitors versus tricyclic antidepressants: a meta-analysis of efficacy and tolerability. *J Affect Disord*. 2000;58(1):19-36.

27. Hageman I, Andersen HS, Jorgensen MB. Post-traumatic stress disorder: a review of psychobiology and pharmacotherapy. *Acta Psychiatr Scand*. 2001;104(6):411-22.

28.   Kessler RC, Soukup J, Davis RB, et al. The use of complementary and alternative therapies to treat anxiety and depression in the United States. *Am J Psychiatry*. 2001;158(2):289-94.

29.   Smith TC, Ryan MA, Smith B, et al. Complementary and alternative medicine use among US Navy and Marine Corps personnel. *BMC Complement Altern Med*. 2007;7:16.

30.   Gordon JS. The White House Commission on Complementary and Alternative Medicine Policy: final report and next steps. *Altern Ther Health Med*. 2002;8(3):28-31.

31.   Agency for Healthcare Research and Quality. Methods Guide for Effectiveness and Comparative Effectiveness Reviews. Rockville, MD: Agency for Healthcare Research and Quality. Available at: http://www.effectivehealthcare.ahrq.gov/index.cfm/search-for-guides-reviews-and-reports/?pageaction=displayproduct&productid=318. Accessed May 31, 2011.

32.   Guyatt GH, Oxman AD, Vist GE, et al. GRADE: an emerging consensus on rating quality of evidence and strength of recommendations. *BMJ*. 2008;336(7650):924-6.

33.   Cohen J. *Statistical power analysis for the behavioral sciences*. 2nd ed Hillsdale, N.J.: L. Erlbaum Associates; 1988.

34.   Kraemer HC, Kupfer DJ. Size of treatment effects and their importance to clinical research and practice. *Biol Psychiatry*. 2006;59(11):990-6.

35.   Short A. Theme and variations on quietness: Relaxation-focused music and imagery in aged care. *Australian Journal of Music Therapy*. 2007;18:39-61.

36.   Carlson JG, Chemtob CM, Rusnak K, et al. Eye movement desensitization and reprocessing (EDMR) treatment for combat-related posttraumatic stress disorder. *J Trauma Stress*. 1998;11(1):3-24.

37.   Marks I, Lovell K, Noshirvani H, et al. Treatment of posttraumatic stress disorder by exposure and/or cognitive restructuring: a controlled study. *Arch Gen Psychiatry*. 1998;55(4):317-25.

38.   Echeburua E, de Corral P, Zubizarreta I, et al. Psychological treatment of chronic posttraumatic stress disorder in victims of sexual aggression. *Behav Modif*. 1997;21(4):433-56.

39.   Taylor S. Outcome Predictors for Three PTSD Treatments: Exposure Therapy, EMDR, and Relaxation Training. *J Cogn Psychother*. 2003;17(2):149-161.

40.   Taylor S, Thordarson DS, Maxfield L, et al. Comparative efficacy, speed, and adverse effects of three ptsd treatments: exposure therapy, emdr, and relaxation training. *J Consult Clin Psychol*. 2003(2):330-8.

41.   Stapleton JA, Taylor S, Asmundson GJ. Effects of three PTSD treatments on anger and guilt: exposure therapy, eye movement desensitization and reprocessing, and relaxation training. *J Trauma Stress*. 2006(1):19-28.

42.   Bormann JE, Thorp S, Wetherell JL, et al. A spiritually based group intervention for combat veterans with posttraumatic stress disorder: feasibility study. *J Holist Nurs*. 2008;26(2):109-16.

43.   Brooks J, Scarano T. Transcendental Meditation in the Treatment of Post-Vietnam Adjustment. *Journal of Counseling and Development*. 1985;64:212-215.

44.   Echeburúa E, de Corral P, Sarasua B, et al. Treatment of acute posttraumatic stress disorder in rape victims: An experimental study. *J Anxiety Disord*. 1996;10(3):185-199.

45.   Hollifield M, Sinclair-Lian N, Warner TD, et al. Acupuncture for posttraumatic stress disorder: a randomized controlled pilot trial. *J Nerv Ment Dis*. 2007;195(6):504-13.

46.   Vaughan K, Armstrong MS, Gold R, et al. A trial of eye movement desensitization compared to image habituation training and applied muscle relaxation in post-traumatic stress disorder. *J Behav Ther Exp Psychiatry*. 1994;25(4):283-91.

47.   Watson CG, Tuorila JR, Vickers KS, et al. The efficacies of three relaxation regimens in the treatment of PTSD in Vietnam war veterans. *J Clin Psychol*; 1997:917-23.

48.   Price C. Body-oriented therapy in sexual abuse recovery: A pilot-test comparison. *J Bodyw Mov Ther*. 2006;10(1):58-64.

49.   Price C. Characteristics of women seeking body-oriented therapy as an adjunct to psychotherapy during recovery from childhood sexual abuse. *J Bodyw Mov Ther*. 2004;8(1):35-42.

50.   Abramowitz EG, Lichtenberg P. A new hypnotic technique for treating combat-related posttraumatic stress disorder: a prospective open study. *Int J Clin Exp Hypn*. 2010;58(3):316-28.

51.   Hossack A, Bentall RP. Elimination of posttraumatic symptomatology by relaxation and visual-kinesthetic dissociation. *J Trauma Stress*. 1996;9(1):99-110.

52.   Bernstein DA, Borkovec TD. *Progressive relaxation training : a manual for the helping professions* Champaign, Ill.: Research Press; 1973.

53.   Ost LG. Applied relaxation: description of a coping technique and review of controlled studies. *Behav Res Ther*. 1987;25(5):397-409.

54.   Rosenthal JZ, Grosswald S, Ross R, et al. Effects of transcendental meditation in veterans of Operation Enduring Freedom and Operation Iraqi Freedom with posttraumatic stress disorder: a pilot study. *Mil Med*. 2011;176(6):626-30.

55.   Schnurr PP, Friedman MJ, Foy DW, et al. Randomized trial of trauma-focused group therapy for posttraumatic stress disorder: results from a department of veterans affairs cooperative study. *Arch Gen Psychiatry*. 2003;60(5):481-9.

56.   Jorm AF, Christensen H, Griffiths KM, et al. Effectiveness of complementary and self-help treatments for anxiety disorders. *Med J Aust*. 2004;181(7 Suppl):S29-46.

57.   Hou WH, Chiang PT, Hsu TY, et al. Treatment effects of massage therapy in depressed people: a meta-analysis. *J Clin Psychiatry*. 2010;71(7):894-901.

58.   Adams E. Brief Overview: Complementary and Alternative Therapies for Post Traumatic Stress Disorder. Veterans Health Administration Office of Patient Care Services Technology Assessment Program. 2009.

59.   Bohlmeijer E, Prenger R, Taal E, et al. The effects of mindfulness-based stress reduction therapy on mental health of adults with a chronic medical disease: a meta-analysis. *J Psychosom Res*. 2010;68(6):539-44.

60.   Grossman P, Niemann L, Schmidt S, et al. Mindfulness-based stress reduction and health benefits. A meta-analysis. *J Psychosom Res*. 2004;57(1):35-43.

61.   Hofmann SG, Sawyer AT, Witt AA, et al. The effect of mindfulness-based therapy on anxiety and depression: A meta-analytic review. *J Consult Clin Psychol*. 2010;78(2):169-83.

62.   Krisanaprakornkit T, Krisanaprakornkit W, Piyavhatkul N, et al. Meditation therapy for anxiety disorders. *Cochrane Database Syst Rev*. 2006(1):CD004998.

63.   Chiesa A. Vipassana meditation: systematic review of current evidence. *J Altern Complement Med*. 2010;16(1):37-46.

64.   Anonymous. World Medical Association. Declaration of Helsinki - Ethical Principles for Medical Research Involving Human Subjects. Available at: http://www.wma.net/en/30publications/10policies/b3/. Accessed May 31, 2011.

65.   Devilly GJ, McFarlane AC. When Wait Lists Are not Feasible, Nothing Is a Thing That Does not Need to Be Done. *J Consult Clin Psychol*. 2009;77(6):1159-1168.

66.   Schnurr PP. The rocks and hard places in psychotherapy outcome research. *J Trauma Stress*. 2007;20(5):779-92.

67.   Cook JA. The challenges faced in the design, conduct and analysis of surgical randomised controlled trials. *Trials*. 2009;10:9.

68.   Schnurr PP, Friedman MJ, Engel CC, et al. Cognitive behavioral therapy for posttraumatic stress disorder in women: a randomized controlled trial. *JAMA: Journal of the American Medical Association*. 2007;297(8):820-830.

69.   Karanicolas PJ, Montori VM, Devereaux PJ, et al. A new 'mechanistic-practical" framework for designing and interpreting randomized trials. *J Clin Epidemiol*. 2009;62(5):479-84.

70.   March J, Kraemer HC, Trivedi M, et al. What have we learned about trial design from NIMH-funded pragmatic trials? *Neuropsychopharmacology*. 2010;35(13):2491-501.

71.   Parmar MK, Ungerleider RS, Simon R. Assessing whether to perform a confirmatory randomized clinical trial. *J Natl Cancer Inst*. 1996;88(22):1645-51.

72.   Smeeding SJ, Bradshaw DH, Kumpfer K, et al. Outcome evaluation of the Veterans Affairs Salt Lake City Integrative Health Clinic for chronic pain and stress-related depression, anxiety, and post-traumatic stress disorder. *J Altern Complement Med.* 2010;16(8):823-35.

73.   Langevin HM, Wayne PM, Macpherson H, et al. Paradoxes in acupuncture research: strategies for moving forward. *Evid Based Complement Alternat Med.* 2011;2011:180805.

74.   Leon AC, Davis LL. Enhancing clinical trial design of interventions for posttraumatic stress disorder. *J Trauma Stress.* 2009;22(6):603-11.

75.   Glasziou P, Chalmers I, Altman DG, et al. Taking healthcare interventions from trial to practice. *BMJ.* 2010;341:c3852.

APPENDIX A. SEARCH STRATEGIES

Step	Goal	Terms	Result[a]
1	**PTSD terms**	Stress Disorders, Traumatic[MeSH] OR stress disorders, post-traumatic[MeSH] OR (post AND traumatic AND stress AND disorder[All Fields]) OR (post-traumatic AND stress AND disorder [All Fields]) OR (post traumatic stress disorder[All Fields]) or (post-traumatic stress disorders[All Fields]) OR ptsd[All Fields] **AND**	1069
2	**Interventions**	Acupuncture Therapy[Mesh:noexpl] OR Acupuncture Analgesia[Mesh] OR Acupuncture, Ear[Mesh] OR Electroacupuncture[Mesh] OR Acupuncture[Mesh] OR Acupressure[Mesh] OR Auriculotherapy[Mesh] OR acupuncture[All Fields] OR (acupuncture[All Fields] AND therapy[All Fields]) OR (acupuncture therapy[All Fields]) OR acupressure[All Fields] OR auriculotherapy[All Fields] OR Mind-Body Therapies[Mesh:noexpl] OR Breathing Exercises[Mesh] OR Hypnosis[Mesh] OR Imagery (Psychotherapy)[Mesh] OR Meditation[Mesh] OR Mental Healing[Mesh] OR Relaxation Therapy[Mesh] OR Tai Ji[Mesh] OR Therapeutic Touch[Mesh] OR Yoga[Mesh] OR Mind-Body Relations, Metaphysical[Mesh] OR breath[All Fields] OR breath[All Fields:expl] OR Complementary Therapies[Mesh:noexpl] OR Holistic Health[Mesh] OR Medicine, East Asian Traditional[Mesh] OR Reflexotherapy[Mesh] OR Spiritual Therapies[Mesh] OR acoustics[MeSH] OR acoustics[All Fields] OR acoustic[All Fields] OR aromatherapy [MeSH] OR sensory[All Fields] OR aromatherapy[All Fields] OR art[MeSH] OR art[All Fields] OR colour[All Fields] OR color[MeSH] OR color[All Fields] OR dance[All Fields] OR music[MeSH] OR music[All Fields] OR play and playthings[MeSH] OR (play AND playthings[All Fields]) OR play and playthings[All Fields] OR play[All Fields] OR sensory art therapies[MeSH] OR reflexotherapy[All Fields] OR craniosacral[All Fields] OR magnet[All Fields] OR light[MeSH] OR light[All Fields] OR feldenkrais[Tiab] OR Alexander[Tiab] OR pilates[All Fields] OR trager[All Fields] OR movement therapeutic[All Fields] OR movement therapies[All Fields] OR movement therapy[All Fields] OR healers[All Fields] OR energy[All Fields] OR therapeutic touch[MeSH] OR (therapeutic[All Fields] AND touch[All Fields]) OR therapeutic touch[All Fields] OR reiki[All Fields]) OR ayurvedic[All Fields] **AND**	83692
3	**Study designs**	Randomized controlled trial[publication type] OR clinical trial[publication type] OR Comparative study[Publication type] OR clinical trials as topic[MeSH] OR (randomized AND controlled AND trial[Tiab]) OR (clinical AND trial[Tiab] OR trial[Tiab:expl] **AND**	13973
4	**Combine results and apply limits**	#1 **AND** #2 **AND** #3 LIMITS: English and Human and Adult	353

[a]Numbers reflect the result of the PubMed search only.

APPENDIX B. STUDY SELECTION FORM

<u>**Citation Screening Instructions**</u>: Turn on revision marks and label each citation with your decision. For studies that you can definitively exclude ($\geq 90\%$), mark with "**E**." For studies that are relevant to CAM for PTSD but not eligible (e.g., a review article), mark with a "**B**" for background. For an article that appears to meet eligibility criteria, mark with "**IN**" for include. We will need to be able to identify comparative studies that appear to meet our eligibility criteria but are excluded because they are not RCTs. Mark these studies with "**F**" for flag, and in the absence of RCTs for a therapy, we will give these studies further scrutiny.

<u>**Inclusion criteria:**</u>

- Study must be an RCT
- Sample population must have diagnosis of PTSD using DSM criteria, validated severity measures (e.g., PTSD Checklist), or clinical diagnosis by a physician
- Sample population is ≥ 19 years of age
- Setting: Patients are recruited from community or outpatient mental health or general medical settings
- Any of the following eligible treatments:
    - Mind-body therapies: Acupuncture, meditation, yoga, deep-breathing exercises, guided imagery, mindfulness-based stress reduction, hypnotherapy, progressive relaxation, qi gong, and tai chi
    - Manipulative and body-based therapies: spinal manipulation, massage therapy
    - Other CAM therapies:
        - Movement-based therapies: Feldenkrais method, Alexander technique, Pilates, Rolfing Structural Integration, and Trager psychophysical integration
    - Manipulation of various energy fields to affect health: magnet therapy, light therapy, qi gong, Reiki, and healing touch
- Comparative studies:
    - Studies that compare an eligible treatment to a control condition—such as usual care (including no treatment, supportive therapy), an attention control, sham intervention, or a waitlist—will be included
    - Studies that compare an eligible treatment to an empirically based treatment such as CBT, PE, or antidepressant medication
- Outcome is reported at ≥ 6 weeks after treatment initiation
- Patients are in acute phase treatment (i.e., not selected for treatment-resistant PTSD)
- Study must be published in a peer-reviewed publication

<u>**Exclusion criteria:**</u>

- Study is a non–English language publication
- Study is conducted outside of North America, Western Europe, Australia, or New Zealand. Studies conducted outside of these countries are unlikely to be applicable to a VA population because of important differences in culture and the health care system.
- Study populations are patients with complicated PTSD: psychosis or acute suicidality

- Studies in which the eligibility criteria <u>require</u> a diagnosis of PTSD comorbid with another mental illness (e.g., PTSD and substance abuse)
- Intervention is used in a continuation phase or maintenance phase
- Excluded interventions:
  - cognitive processing therapy
  - eye movement desensitization and reprocessing (EMDR)
  - generic counseling
  - life review therapy
  - psychoeducational therapy
  - social support or supportive therapy
  - standard psychodynamic therapy
  - "third wave" cognitive and behavioral therapies: mindfulness-based cognitive therapy, dialectical behavioral therapy, and acceptance and commitment therapy
  - other treatments that are a direct extension of an established conventional therapy (e.g., Imagery Rehearsal Therapy)
  - incident stress debriefing, psychological debriefing
  - trauma-focused therapy
  - present-focused therapy
  - seeking-safety treatment
  - relaxation therapy used as a control arm or not described in sufficient detail to understand the key components

APPENDIX C. SAMPLE DATA EXTRACTION FORM

Study Information (Author/Year/EN#): _____

Other linked studies? (1) No   (2) Yes: _____

1. **Study objective**: _____
    _____

2. **Study location (1-4 sites):** ☐ NA

    a. Location 1: City_____ Country:_____
    b. Location 2: City_____ Country:_____
    c. Location 3: City_____ Country:_____
    d. Location 4: City_____ Country:_____

3. **Study location (If > 4 sites):** ☐ NA Sites (#): _____ Countries/regions(#): _____

    Names of regions (e.g. Western Europe) _____

4. **Treatment setting (all that apply)**:
    (1) Mental Health   (2) Gen. Medical   (3) Non-Medical   (4) NR

5. **VA settings**:   (1) Yes   (2) No   (3) Mixed   (4) NR

6. **Active duty military settings**: (1) Yes   (2) No   (3) Mixed   (4) NR

7. **Academic affiliation**:   (1) Yes   (2) No   (3) Mixed   (4) NR

8. **Study design**:
    (1) Patient level RCT   (2) Non-randomized controlled trial (3) Cross-over trial
    (4) Prospective cohort study   (5) Case Series   (6) Other: _____

9. **Subject recruitment (all that apply)**: (1) Screening   (2) Clinician referral
    (3) Advertisement (paid)   (4) Other (list):_____   (5) NR

Characteristics of the participants   1. Total enrolled: _____

Characteristic	Total Enrolled	Intervention	Control
2. Mean age (SD)			
3. Sex: Men (n)			
4. Sex: Women (n)			
5. Race: White (n)			
6. Race: African American (n)			
7. Race: Latino (n)			
8. Race: Asian (n)			
9a. Mean (SD) education (years) or			
9b. ≥ High school education (n)			
10. Mean (SD) PTSD severity: _____			
11. Mean (SD) Functional status: _____			
12. Mean (SD) Years since trauma			

1. **Eligibility Criteria**:

    a. Diagnosis: (1) DSM3R   (2) DSMIV   (3) ICD   (4) Clinical-nonstandardized

        (5) Severity measure (e.g., PCL)   (6) Patient self-reports diagnosis

    b. Trauma exposure (all that apply): (1) Combat   (2) Natural disaster

        (3) Rape/sexual assault   (4) Childhood abuse   (5) Physical assault   (6) Transportation

        accident (7) Other_____

    c. Age range: _____

    d. Suspend other psychological treatment: (1) Yes   (2) No

    e. Keep psychotropic medications stable: (1) Yes   (2) No

    f. Other 1: _____

    g. Other 2:_____

2. **Exclusion Criteria**:

    a. Alcohol or substance abuse: (1) Yes   (2) No   (3) Not reported

    b. Psychotic disorder: (1) Yes   (2) No   (3) Not reported

    c. Reason 1: _____   Reason 2:_____

    d. Reason 3:_____   Reason 4: _____

Intervention

1. Intervention:_____

2. Sessions planned (#):_____   Mean (SD) Sessions delivered:_____

3. Duration planned (minutes/session): _____

4. Discipline: (1) Physician   (2) PhD MH professional (3) Masters train MH professional

[All that apply] (4) Physical therapist   (5) Chiropractor (6) Trained research assistant

            (7) Trained acupuncturist (8) Other: _____

5. Mean years of experience (SD):_____

6. Study-specific training: _____

7. Intervention components:

    a. Component 1:_____ (allowed | given)

    b. Component 2:_____ (allowed | given)

    c. Component 3:_____(allowed | given)

    d. Component 4:_____ (allowed | given)

    e. Component 5:_____ (allowed | given)

8. Is the intervention described in sufficient detail for a trained practitioner to replicate?

    (1) Yes (2) No

Comparator (If active comparator choose PE or CPT > EMDR>Other)

9. Basic descriptor: (1) Usual Care   (2) Sham   (3) Attention Control   (4) Waitlist

    (5) CPT (6) Exposure therapy   (7) Other: _____

10. Sessions planned (#):_____   Mean (SD) Sessions delivered:_____

11. Duration planned (minutes/session):_____

12. Clinician same discipline as for the intervention? (1) Yes   (2) No (3) NR

13. Comparator Components:

    f. Component 1: _____ (allowed | given)

    g. Component 2: _____ (allowed | given)

    h. Component 3: _____ (allowed | given)

    i. Component 4: _____ (allowed | given)

    j. Component 4: _____ (allowed | given)

14. If 3-arm trial, other comparator: _____

Outcomes

1. Subjects randomized:_____   Number Analyzed:_____

2. Time 1 f/u (weeks): _____   Time 1 f/u (n): _____

3. Time 2 f/u (weeks): _____   Time 2 f/u (n): _____

4. Other time points reported: (1) No   (2) Yes (weeks): a. ____   b. ____   c.___

5. Response definition (% change):_____

6. Remission definition:_____

7. Symptom measure 1: _____ □ Self-report   □ Interviewer rated

8. Symptom measure 2: _____ □ Self-report   □ Interviewer rated

9. HRQOL measure: _____ □ Self-report   □ Interviewer rated

10. Outcome measure 4: _____ □ Self-report   □ Interviewer rated

11. Adherence measured: (1) sessions completed   (2) homework   (3) both

12. Outcomes reported as dichotomous results – time point 1 (weeks):_____
    OR □ No dichotomous results reported

Outcome	NR	Intervention		Comparator	
		Events (n)	At risk (n)	Events (n)	At risk (n)
AE: Discontinuation					
AE: Any					
Clinical response					
Clinical remission					
Completer					

13. Time point 2 Results (weeks):_____OR □ No time point 2 dichotomous results

Outcome	NR	Intervention		Comparator	
		Events (n)	At risk (n)	Events (n)	At risk (n)
AE: Discontinuation					
AE: Any					
Clinical response					
Clinical remission					
Completer					

14. Continuous results – time point 1 (weeks)_____ give mean (SD) or mean (95% CI; x to y)
    □ No continuous results reported

Outcome	Intervention baseline	Comparator baseline	Intervention followup	Int "n"	Comparator followup	Comp "n"	F/U Code
Adherence	NA	NA					
Sx score 1							
Sx Score 2							
HRQOL							
Patient satisfaction							
Social functioning							

F/U Code: U=Unadjusted Mean (e.g., ANOVA); A=Adjusted mean (e.g, ANCOVA); C1=Change score for treatment arm (T2-T1); C2=Change score for treatment arm (T1-T2); D1 = Difference in means between groups at followup (intervention – comparator, e.g., estimate from mixed model); D2 = Difference in means between groups at followup (comparator - intervention); P=only a p value given (record p value in the Intervention f/u field)

15. Continuous results – time point 2 (weeks):_____ give mean (SD) or mean (95% CI; x to y)

□ No Dichotomous results reported at time point 2

Outcome	Intervention baseline	Comparator baseline	Intervention followup	Int "n"	Comparator followup	Comp "n"	F/U Code
Adherence	NA	NA					
Sx score 1							
Sx Score 2							
HRQOL							
Patient satisfaction							
Social functioning							

F/U Code: U=Unadjusted Mean (e.g., ANOVA); A=Adjusted mean (e.g, ANCOVA); C1=Change score for treatment arm (T2-T1); C2=Change score for treatment arm (T1-T2); D1 = Difference in means between groups at followup (intervention – comparator, e.g., estimate from mixed model); D2 = Difference in means between groups at followup (comparator - intervention); P=only a p value given (record p value in the Intervention f/u field)

APPENDIX D. CRITERIA USED IN QUALITY ASSESSMENT

General Instructions:
For each risk of bias item, rate as "Yes," "No," or "Unclear." After considering each of the quality items, give the study an overall quality rating of good, fair or poor.

<u>Detailed Quality Items:</u>
If an item is rated as "No," describe why in the comments column.

1. *Randomization adequate?* Was the allocation sequence adequately generated? **Yes/No/Unclear**
2. *Allocation concealment adequate?* Was allocation adequately concealed? **Yes/No/Unclear**
3. *Incomplete outcome data adequately addressed?* **Yes/No/Unclear**
   Consider Attrition bias: Were there systematic differences between groups in withdrawals from a study or high overall loss to followup? (Even small differences could be important when rates are low.) Were subjects excluded from the analysis – if so, were the exclusions sensible?
4. *Subjects Blinded?* Were subjects blind to treatment assignment? **Yes/No/Unclear**
5. *Outcome assessor blinded?* (This may be recorded separately for each critically important outcome.) Were Outcome assessors blind to treatment assignment? **Yes/No/Unclear**
6. *Provider (treating clinician) blinded?* Were providers blind to treatment assignment? **Yes/No/Unclear**
7. *All outcomes reported?* Are reports of the study free of suggestion of selective outcome reporting (systematic differences between reported and unreported findings)? **Yes/No/Unclear**
8. *Intention-to-treat analysis?* All eligible patients that were randomized are included in analysis; note- mixed models and survival analyses are in general ITT **Yes/No/Unclear**
9. *Adequate power for main effects?* **Yes** (if power analysis or sample size calculation given and recruitment met needs or if post-hoc power calculation shows adequate power)/**No** (did not meet projected sample size needs) /**Unclear** (no power or sample size calculation given)
10. *Other Selection bias?* Were there methods that could lead to differences or were there systematic differences observed in baseline characteristics and prognostic factors of the groups compared?(e.g., failure of randomization): **Yes/No/Unclear**
11. *Comparable groups maintained?* (Includes crossovers, adherence, and contamination.) Consider issues of crossover (e.g., from one intervention to another), adherence (major differences in adherence to the interventions being compared), contamination (e.g., some members of control group get intervention) **Yes/No/Unclear**
12. *Lack of Performance bias?* Were there no important systematic differences in the care that was provided, other than the intervention of interest? **Yes/No/Unclear**
13. *Lack of Measurement bias?* Were the measures used reliable and valid – and therefore, "yes" no important measurement bias? **Yes/No/Unclear**
14. *Absence of Detection bias?* Were there systematic differences between groups in how outcomes are determined? If no systematic differences answer "yes" – no important detection bias. **Yes/No/Unclear**
15. *Was there the absence of potential important conflict of interest?* The focus here is financial conflict of interest. Therefore if no financial conflict of interest (e.g. funded by government or foundation and authors do not have financial relationships with drug/device manufacturer), then answer "yes." **Yes/No/Unclear**

Overall rating

Please assign each study an overall quality rating of "Good," "Fair," or "Poor" based on the following definitions:

A "**Good**" study has the least bias, and results are considered valid. A good study has a clear description of the population, setting, interventions, and comparison groups; uses a valid approach to allocate patients to alternative treatments; has a low dropout rate; and uses appropriate means to prevent bias, measure outcomes, and analyze and report results.

A "**Fair**" study is susceptible to some bias but probably not enough to invalidate the results. The study may be missing information, making it difficult to assess limitations and potential problems. As the fair-quality category is broad, studies with this rating vary in their strengths and weaknesses. The results of some fair-quality studies are possibly valid, while others are probably valid.

A "**Poor**" rating indicates significant bias that may invalidate the results. These studies have serious errors in design, analysis, or reporting; have large amounts of missing information; or have discrepancies in reporting. The results of a poor-quality study are at least as likely to reflect flaws in the study design as to indicate true differences between the compared interventions.

APPENDIX E. PEER REVIEW COMMENTS/AUTHOR RESPONSES

Reviewer	Comment	Response
Question 1: Are the objectives, scope, and methods for this review clearly described?		
1	Yes	Acknowledged
2	Yes	Acknowledged
3	Yes - This is an excellent review and evidence synthesis.	Thank you.
4	Yes	Acknowledged
5	Yes – This was a clearly and well-defined project. The authors are to be congratulated on the organization of the report which made for easy reading.	Thank you.
	This reviewer would appreciate a formal definition of CAM (if there is such) early in the introductory material.	This definition is provided on the first page of the Executive Summary and in the background section of the Introduction of the report.
	Also, I realize that natural products such as nutritional supplements were excluded from review, but there was no convincing rationale for this decision. Given the paucity of information from other CAM approaches, it might be worth reconsidering this decision.	The decision to exclude nutritional supplements was made by the stakeholders, not the research team.
6	Yes	Acknowledged
Question 2: Is there any indication of bias in our synthesis of the evidence?		
1	No	Acknowledged
2	Yes – The exclusion criteria listed on p 12-13 show a clear bias toward western medicine centric locations. Given the paucity of studies, inclusion of a wider selection of studies particularly from countries where CAM is more common would be warranted. This would also involve non-English language publications.	The reviewer raises a valid point. Our conceptual framework was to review settings and subjects similar to the VA and Veterans—thus the focus on studies conducted in the U.S. and economically similar countries. Our staff is not resourced to include non-English publications. We note this limitation in the discussion.
3	No	Acknowledged
4	No	Acknowledged
5	No	Acknowledged
6	Yes - There is no evidence of intentional bias. The authors have done a very fair job of reporting the evidence. However, I believe the selection criteria may have limited what can be learned from the existing evidence, and therefore, have created an unintentional bias in the conclusions.	See response to Question 7, Reviewer 6

Reviewer	Comment	Response
Question 3: Are there any studies of interest to the VA that we have overlooked?		
1	Yes Rosenthal, et al. (2011). Military Medicine, 176:626-630	Thank you for making us aware of this article. Although it was published after our literature search date (Dec 22, 2010) and thus excluded from our formal literature synthesis, we now include a description of this study in our Results section, Key Question 4.
2	Yes - see comments above on excluded studies. since PTSD is commonly comorbid with substance abuse, exclusion of studies requiring both diagnoses limits applicability of findings The listing of the references for the excluded studies is a plus, as the reader can draw their own conclusions. Shore 2004 is missing from that list. Management of Operation Iraqi Freedom and Operation Enduring Freedom veterans in a Veterans Health Administration chiropractic clinic: a case series. Lisi AJ. Journal of Rehabilitation Research & Development. 47(1):1-6, 2010	Acknowledged Shore 2004 is included in the excluded studies table in Appendix F. Thank you for bringing this article to our attention. However, it does not meet our inclusion criteria since PTSD diagnosis was not a study inclusion criteria, nor was change in PTSD a reported outcome.
3	No – none that I am aware of, but this is not my field	Acknowledged
4	No - none that I am aware of	Acknowledged
5	No	Acknowledged
6	Yes - There is an RCT of mindfulness meditation by Barbara Niles that is relevant. I believe that the authors attempted to get a copy of the paper but could not for some reason. However, the trial was well-done and positive, so it would be helpful to try to include it if at all possible.	We have obtained a prepublication draft of this manuscript but do not include it in the current report since our literature review strategy stipulates that included studies be published in peer-reviewed journals.
Question 4: Are there any clinical performance measures, programs, quality improvement measures, patient care services, or conferences that will be directly affected by this report? If so, please provide detail.		
1	The findings of this report will be used while designing demonstration projects in the field, in an attempt to address some of the methodological limitations identified in the report.	Acknowledged
2	None	
3	No, the evidence base is too limited	Acknowledged

Efficacy of Complementary and Alternative Medicine Therapies for Posttraumatic Stress Disorder

Reviewer	Comment	Response
4	The finding of limitations of current scientific evidence to review and the recommendation for investment in adequately powered trials may affect and push such research trials. This could result in positive results for patient care services.	Acknowledged
5	In order to facilitate health services research in this area I the VA, it would be great to have some procedure codes that could be universally adopted that would capture various CAM approaches.	Thank you for this suggestion. We have added it to our Future Research section.
6	None that I can think of	Acknowledged
Question 5: Please provide any recommendations on how this report can be revised to more directly address or assist implementation needs.		
1	We would like to immediately be able to provide the draft version of this report to our evaluation team from the University of Rochester, who will be designing the evaluation structure of our demonstration projects. Please advise if this is possible, or if not, when the report can be available to them. This work will begin very soon, so this is time sensitive.	Acknowledged
2	None	
3	This is an excellent report and I have only a few suggestions for how to revise it to improve it.	Thank you.
	1. Page 15. The description of the data synthesis is somewhat difficult to understand, especially the last couple of lines. It may not be to experts in this field however. It would be nice if this could be a little clearer.	We revised the data synthesis section to more clearly describe the standardized mean difference.
	2. I think it would be very helpful to include the quality ratings on Table 4 as well as a brief sentence or 2 interpreting the important findings in the study rather than relying on the reader either understanding the measurements or referring back to them to understand what the findings mean.	We added the quality ratings for each study in Table 4. Outcomes are summarized in text. There was not adequate space to summarize the results narratively in the table.
	3. On page 26, clarify that the study by Echeburua is a study of CBT/coping not of relaxation (if I understand it correctly)	Echeburúa and colleagues conducted a comparative effectiveness study of relaxation training (progressive muscle relaxation; PMR) to an intervention that included cognitive behavioral therapy, coping, and PMR. We have updated the description of the study and Table 4 to better describe the two treatment arms.

Reviewer	Comment	Response
3 (Cont'd.)	4. Page 41 last paragraph----why so much discussion about Vujanovic and their thoughts. is there data on mindfulness to support this contention? Does it deserve this much space in this report if no data and only opinion?	We agree. In the final report, we have markedly streamlined this portion of the discussion.
4	None	
5	None	
6	Given the widespread use of CAM across the VA, clinicians, researchers, and administrators may find the report to be useful in helping them understand the evidence base on CAM for PTSD.	Thank you.
Question 6: Please provide us with contact details of any additional individuals/stakeholders who should be made aware of this report.		
1	Dr. Madhu Agarwal, info in VA Outlook	Thank you. We will be sure Dr. Agarwal is made aware of the report.
2	None	
3	None	
4	None	
5	None	
6	None	
Question 7: Please write additional suggestions or comments below. If applicable, please indicate the page and line numbers from the draft report.		
1	p.10, I believe that the number who have deployed in the current conflicts is closer to 2.2 million	Thank you for this comment. The report introduction now reflects an estimated 2.2 million deployed.
	Overall, I am not sure why nonscientific "energy therapies" are included with movement based therapies, but since you didn't find any efficacy, I guess it doesn't matter.	We included energy therapies and movement therapies within the same category, consistent with NCCAM's classification system for these modalities.
2	None	
3	I would like to identify some features of this report that are very helpful in understanding this literature synthesis and might be applicable to other ESP reports. These include:	Thank you!
	1. Table 1 is excellent and a nice model for our reports. It is very clear.	
	2. Table 5 is really nice. Very helpful.	
	3. Table 9 is great! again, an interpretation of the findings might be helpful to the less knowledgeable reader	

Reviewer	Comment	Response
4	None	
5	It would be terrific if there could be a parallel review of CAM therapies related to major depression and some of the non-PTSD anxiety disorders. These conditions tend to be comorbid with PTSD as well as share some symptomatology. More importantly, there are many treatments that are identical for these conditions and PTSD (e.g., SSRI's, sleep medications), so it would make sense that some CAM approaches that are successful for these conditions might also be successful for PTSD. Thus, it would be extremely useful to have such a review. In addition to the efficacy results, such a review could also point to methodological considerations as well as touch on patient acceptability.	We thank the reviewer for this suggestion. This supplementary report has already been commissioned, is underway, and should be available in the fall of 2011.
	It would be helpful to include a brief description of the AHRQ study quality methods in the text.	A brief description of the AHRQ quality methods is presented in the Methods section under Quality Assessment.
	I would remove the statement on page 4 (and elsewhere in the text) that lower standards of evidence may be applicable when CAM treatments are offered as adjuncts to conventional, evidence-based PTSD therapies. Even in the context of an add-on therapy, it is important to conduct high quality studies.	We appreciate this reviewer's comment. The Future Research section has been revised substantially and this statement has been omitted from the discussion.
	Page 6: It is problematic to omit mention of veterans of previous wars (e.g., Persian Gulf, Vietnam, etc.). Vietnam veterans are by far the most numerous in the VA system, so they and other previous war era veterans should be included in this introductory paragraph.	Thank you for this suggestion. We have expanded the introductory text to acknowledge Veterans of all service eras.
	At some point in the paper (perhaps when discussing future research?), it may be a good idea to discuss some of the complexities of PTSD research. These include a variety of traumas (e.g., natural disasters, combat, rape, etc) which may respond differentially to treatments, time since trauma (which may impact on symptom severity), and comorbidity (both psychiatric and medical).	We thank the reviewer for this observation. A full discussion of the complexities of PTSD research was beyond the scope of this report, but we have highlighted some key challenges and referred the reader to more in-depth discussions.
	Thank you for the opportunity to review this report. I hope these comments will be useful to increase the report's utility.	Thank you!

Reviewer	Comment	Response
6	The study team did a very careful job in preparing this document. The writing is clear and thorough. However, I feel that the document could be more useful if the authors made several revisions.	Thank you.
	The approach, which is very strict about inclusion and exclusion, would be a better fit with a literature that was more evolved, in which there were more studies and more definitive studies. With such a small and underdeveloped literature, it would have been informative to include a broader range of studies. Doing so could have influenced the conclusions about what appears to be promising—even if those conclusions were not definitive.	The research team understands this observation by the reviewer. However, our conceptual framework was to review settings and subjects similar to the VA and Veterans for ease of implementation if there was strong evidence for a therapy.
	The most important example of this concerns the exclusion of studies that used relaxation as a comparison treatment but did not provide an adequate description of the relaxation protocol. At least a couple of these studies (Carlson and Marks) found that relaxation was less effective than treatments recommended in the VA/DoD PTSD practice guideline. The Marks study, which was published in the Archives of General Psychiatry, would be considered to be at least good or better quality. Although the statement about relaxation on p.29 is not very favorable, by not reviewing studies such as Carlson and Marks, it might appear that relaxation is an intervention in need of evaluation. However, its performance in the 3 studies reviewed and these 2 additional studies suggests that it may not have promise. Of course, this conclusion needs to be tempered by the absence of detail about what study participants actually received. However, the information could be presented to readers, with this caveat mentioned.	We have added text to the Limitation section to acknowledge this important point.
	I do not know how the criteria that caused other studies to be excluded might have affected the results. The point is a more inclusive review that extracted more information from the existing literature could provide useful guidance about future directions.	Acknowledged

Reviewer	Comment	Response
6 (cont.)	I also recommend that the authors revise content in the section on Future Directions (p. 4), and carry these revisions into the more extensive summary on pp. 41-45. Using the p. 4 content as a reference:	
	• The first paragraph discusses usual care and no care interventions as if they are the same, when they are not. The inferences drawn from a usual care design are different and stronger than the inferences drawn from a no care design.	The text has been revised to refer to no care (waitlist) controls.
	• The second paragraph suggests that "evidence of benefit from less rigorous trial designs may be sufficient" for CAM treatments for PTSD that are los costs, responsive to patient preferences, and have few adverse effects. There is nothing in the review to support this suggestion. Low cost, low risk intervention that patients like may not be a good use of resources at a system level and could interfere with the delivery of effective care. Except for the patient-centeredness of this suggestion, I do not think it fits with VA's model of quality care. Furthermore, why would a lower standard of evidence be a good idea in any case?	The Future Research section has been revised substantially, and the endorsement of lower quality evidence and discussion of costs have been removed.
	• The third paragraph concludes that medication, acupuncture, relaxation, and mind-body interventions are feasible and acceptable to patients and "may hold promise as adjunctive of monotherapies for PTSD." Based on the literature review, it is not possible to draw such a broad, if suggestive, conclusion about the benefits of monotherapy and adjunctive therapy for all of these treatments. None of them were tested in both formats. Furthermore, the tone of the conclusion does not fit with the summary of the evidence on p. 29 or the table on pp. 39-40. Findings based on small, primarily poor or fair quality studies (for which the strength of evidence for all treatment/comparator combinations is rated as low or insufficient except for acupuncture), are not an adequate basis for concluding that the interventions tested may be promising. There is only one good-quality study, of acupuncture as monotherapy (although study participants were allowed to use medication and receive supportive therapy).	We agree that the conclusions were overly broad. The conclusions have been modified and reflect the concerns raised by this reviewer.

Reviewer	Comment	Response
6 (cont.)	The recommendations for future research should include recommendations about completeness of reporting and fidelity monitoring, both of which are problems in the literature reviewed. Testing CAM interventions as monotherapy versus adjunctive therapies also would be helpful. There could be an argument that CAM as monotherapy should use EBT as a comparator given the strength of data now available for the EBTs.	Recommendations about fidelity monitoring and completeness of outcomes reporting have been specifically addressed in the revised Future Research section.
	The content on mindfulness on pp. 41-42 seems out of place in a section on limitations. This content is not about the limitations of the report.	We concur and now omit this content from the limitations section.
	I recommend that the authors standardize the level of detail provided about different studies. For example, in the section on relaxation (pp. 26-29), F and p-values are reported for the Watson study, p-values are reported for the Vaughn study, and Ms and SDs are reported for the Echeburúa study.	Thank you for this observation. We have attempted to standardize this section.
	I also recommend that the authors try to reduce jargon when possible. Sentences like the 3rd bullet on 0. 29 are difficult to understand.	Thank you for this observation. We have attempted this where possible.

APPENDIX F. EXCLUDED STUDIES

All studies listed below were reviewed in their full-text version and excluded for the reason indicated. An alphabetical reference list follows the table.

Reference	Population not PTSD	Setting not outpatient, PC, MH, or community	Intervention not eligible CAM treatment	Control or comparator not eligible condition	Location not US/Europe/New Zealand/Australia	Language not English	Not peer reviewed/not primary data
Bob, 2004 (1220)	X						
Branstrom, 2010 (43)	X						
Bryant, 2005 (243)	X						
Cardena, 2000 (732)							X
Carlson, 1998 (259)			X				
Carter, 2006 (402)							X
Descilo, 2010 (357)					X		
Dunn, 2009 (950)	X						
Echeburúa 1997 (260)			X				
Frueh, 2007 (1388)			X				
Gordon, 2004 (313)				X			
Hiley-Young, 1990 (1874)			X				
Kraft, 2010 (490)	X						
Marks, 1998 (258)			X				
Nakamura, 2010 (748)	X						
Peeke, 2002 (483)							X
Salerno, 2005 (1312)		X					
Shore, 2004 (1793)	X						
Short, 2007 (1315)	X						
Spira, 2006 (758)	X						
Stapleton, 2006 (401)			X				
Stapleton, 2007 (1057)			X				
Tacón, 2009 (1137)		X					
Tarrier, 1999 (257)			X				
Taylor, 2003 (425)			X				
Taylor, 2003 (1157)			X				
Trzepacz, 2004 (1056)			X				
Valentine, 2001 (1522)						X	
Waelde, 2008 (954)	X						

LIST OF EXCLUDED STUDIES

Bob P. Psychophysiology of hypnotic abreaction. Homeost Health Dis. 2004;43(2):109-111.

Branstrom R, Kvillemo P, Brandberg Y, et al. Self-report mindfulness as a mediator of psychological well-being in a stress reduction intervention for cancer patients--a randomized study. Ann Behav Med. 2010;39(2):151-61.

Bryant RA, Moulds ML, Guthrie RM, et al. The additive benefit of hypnosis and cognitive-behavioral therapy in treating acute stress disorder. J Consult Clin Psychol. 2005;73(2):334-40.

Cardena E. Hypnosis in the treatment of trauma: A promising, but not fully supported, efficacious intervention. Int J Clin Exp Hypn. 2000;48(2):225-238.

Carlson JG, Chemtob CM, Rusnak K, et al. Eye movement desensitization and reprocessing (EDMR) treatment for combat-related posttraumatic stress disorder. J Trauma Stress. 1998;11(1):3-24.

Carter JJ. Evaluation of a multi-component yoga intervention as adjunct to psychiatric treatment for Vietnam veterans with posttraumatic stress disorder (PTSD): A randomized controlled trial (RCT). controlled-trials.com; 2006.

Descilo T, Vedamurtachar A, Gerbarg PL, et al. Effects of a yoga breath intervention alone and in combination with an exposure therapy for post-traumatic stress disorder and depression in survivors of the 2004 South-East Asia tsunami. Acta Psychiatr Scand; 2010:289-300.

Dunn AS, Passmore SR, Burke J, et al. A cross-sectional analysis of clinical outcomes following chiropractic care in veterans with and without post-traumatic stress disorder. Mil Med. 2009;174(6):578-583.

Echeburua E, de Corral P, Zubizarreta I, et al. Psychological treatment of chronic posttraumatic stress disorder in victims of sexual aggression. Behav Modif. 1997;21(4):433-56.

Frueh BC, Monnier J, Yim E, et al. A randomized trial of telepsychiatry for post-traumatic stress disorder. J Telemed Telecare. 2007;13(3):142-147.

Gordon JS, Staples JK, Blyta A, et al. Treatment of posttraumatic stress disorder in postwar Kosovo high school students using mind-body skills groups: a pilot study. J Trauma Stress. 2004;17(2):143-7.

Hiley-Young B. Facilitating Cognitive-Emotional Congruence in Anxiety Disorders During Self-Determined Cognitive Change: An Integrative Model J Cogn Psychother. 1990;4(2):225-236.

Kraft K, Telles S. Yoga practice may be useful after post-traumatic stress. Focus on Alternative and Complementary Therapies. 2010;15(3):255-256.

Marks I, Lovell K, Noshirvani H, et al. Treatment of posttraumatic stress disorder by exposure and/or cognitive restructuring: a controlled study. Arch Gen Psychiatry. 1998;55(4):317-25.

Nakamura Y, Lipschitz DL, Landward R, et al. Two sessions of sleep-focused mind-body bridging improve self-reported symptoms of sleep and PTSD in veterans: A pilot randomized controlled trial. J Psychosom Res. 2010.

Peeke PM, Frishett S. The role of complementary and alternative therapies in women's mental health. Primary Care - Clinics in Office Practice. 2002;29(1):183-197.

Salerno N. The Use of Hypnosis in the Treatment of Post-traumatic Stress Disorder in a Female Correctional Setting. Australian Journal of Clinical & Experimental Hypnosis. 2005;33(1):74-81.

Shore A. Long-term effects of energetic healing on symptoms of psychological depression and self-perceived stress. Altern Ther Health Med 2004;10(3):42-8.

Short A. Theme and variations on quietness: Relaxation-focused music and imagery in aged care. Australian Journal of Music Therapy. 2007;18:39-61.

Spira JL, Pyne JM, Wiederhold B, et al. Virtual reality and other experiential therapies for combat-related posttraumatic stress disorder. Primary Psychiatry. 2006;13(3):58-64.

Stapleton JA, Taylor S, Asmundson GJ. Effects of three PTSD treatments on anger and guilt: exposure therapy, eye movement desensitization and reprocessing, and relaxation training. J Trauma Stress. 2006(1):19-28.

Stapleton JA, Taylor S, Asmundson GJG. Efficacy of various treatments for PTSD in battered women: Case studies. J Cogn Psychother. 2007;21(1):91-102.

Tacón AM, McComb J. Mindful exercise, quality of life, and survival: A mindfulness-based exercise program for women with breast cancer. The Journal of Alternative and Complementary Medicine. 2009;15(1):41-46.

Tarrier N, Pilgrim H, Sommerfield C, et al. A randomized trial of cognitive therapy and imaginal exposure in the treatment of chronic posttraumatic stress disorder. J Consult Clin Psychol. 1999;67(1):13-8.

Taylor S, Thordarson DS, Maxfield L, et al. Comparative efficacy, speed, and adverse effects of three ptsd treatments: exposure therapy, emdr, and relaxation training. J Consult Clin Psychol. 2003(2):330-8.

Taylor S. Outcome Predictors for Three PTSD Treatments: Exposure Therapy, EMDR, and Relaxation Training. J Cogn Psychother. 2003;17(2):149-161.

Trzepacz AM, Luiselli JK. Efficacy of Stress Inoculation Training in a Case of Posttraumatic Stress Disorder (PTSD) Secondary to Emergency Gynecological Surgery. Clinical Case Studies. 2004;3(1):83-92.

Valentine PV, Smith TE. Evaluating traumatic incident reduction therapy with female inmates: a randomized controlled clinical trial. Research on Social Work Practice. 2001;11(1):40-52.

Waelde LC, Uddo M, Marquett R, et al. A pilot study of meditation for mental health workers following Hurricane Katrina. J Trauma Stress. 2008;21(5):497-500.

APPENDIX G. GLOSSARY

Acupuncture

A family of procedures involving stimulation of anatomical points on the body by a variety of techniques. American practices of acupuncture incorporate medical traditions from China, Japan, Korea, and other countries. The acupuncture technique that has been most studied scientifically involves penetrating the skin with thin, solid, metallic needles that are manipulated by the hands or by electrical stimulation.

Alexander technique

A movement therapy that uses guidance and education about ways to improve posture and movement. The intent is to teach a person how to use muscles more efficiently in order to improve the overall functioning of the body.

Ayurvedic medicine

A system of medicine that originated in India thousands of years ago. Ayurveda is based on theories of health and illness and on ways to prevent, manage, or treat health problems. A chief aim of Ayurvedic practices is to cleanse the body of substances that can cause disease, and this is believed to help reestablish harmony and balance.

Biofeedback

A technique that uses simple electronic devices to teach clients how to consciously regulate bodily functions, such as breathing, heart rate, and blood pressure, in order to improve overall health. Biofeedback is used to reduce stress, eliminate headaches, recondition injured muscles, control asthmatic attacks, and relieve pain.

Chiropractic care

A type of care that involves the adjustment of the spine and joints to influence the body's nervous system and natural defense mechanisms to alleviate pain and improve general health. It is primarily used to treat back problems, headaches, nerve inflammation, muscle spasms, and other injuries and traumas.

Cognitive behavioral therapy (CBT)

A psychotherapeutic approach that aims to solve problems concerning dysfunctional emotions, behaviors, and cognitions through a goal-oriented, systematic procedure. The term is used in diverse ways to designate behavior therapy, cognitive therapy, or therapy based on a combination of the two.

Cognitive processing therapy (CPT)

A cognitive behavioral therapy for PTSD and related conditions. CPT conceptualizes PTSD as a disorder of "nonrecovery" in which erroneous beliefs about the causes and consequences of traumatic events produce strong negative emotions and prevent accurate processing of the trauma memory and natural emotions emanating from the event.

Complementary and alternative medicine (CAM)

A group of diverse medical and health care systems, practices, and products that are not generally considered part of conventional medicine. Complementary medicine is used together with conventional medicine, and alternative medicine is used in place of conventional medicine.

Energy therapy

A practice that involves channeling of energy through the hands of a practitioner into the patient's body to restore a normal energy balance and health. It is often used in conjunction with alternative and conventional medical treatments.

Eye movement desensitization and reprocessing (EMDR)

A form of psychotherapy developed to resolve symptoms resulting from disturbing and unresolved life experiences. EMDR uses a structured approach to address past, present, and future aspects of disturbing memories.

Exposure therapy

A type of behavior therapy in which the patient confronts a feared situation, object, thought, or memory. Sometimes exposure therapy involves reliving a traumatic experience in a controlled, therapeutic environment. The goal is to reduce the distress, physical or emotional, felt in certain situations.

Feldenkrais

A movement therapy that uses a method of education in physical coordination and movement. The intent is to help the person become more aware of how the body moves through space and to improve physical functioning.

Frontalis muscle tension

Tension or pain in the muscle tissues that run vertically on the forehead.

Guided imagery

A mind-body approach involving a series of relaxation techniques followed by visualization of detailed images, usually calm and peaceful in nature. If used for treatment, the individual will visualize their body free of the specific problem or condition.

Health-related quality of life (HRQOL)

Aspects of overall quality of life that can be clearly shown to affect health—either physical or mental.

Image habituation training (IHT)

A form of exposure therapy that involves the patient in generating verbal descriptions of the traumatic event and recording these onto an audiotape.

Intent-to-treat analysis

A method of analyzing results of a randomized controlled trial that includes in the analysis all cases that should have received a treatment regimen but for some reason did not. All cases allocated to each arm of the trial are analyzed together as representing that treatment arm, regardless of whether they received or completed the prescribed regimen.

Magnet therapy

An approach that applies a magnetic field to the body for purported health benefits including pain control. Magnets in products such as magnetic patches and disks, shoe insoles, bracelets, and mattress pads are used for pain in the foot, wrist, back, and other parts of the body.

Manipulative and body-based practices

Practices that focus primarily on the structures and systems of the body, including the bones and joints, soft tissues, and circulatory and lymphatic systems. Two commonly used therapies in this category are spinal manipulation and massage therapy.

Mantram

A sound, syllable, word, or group of words used in meditation practice to focus attention and achieve a state of greater calmness, physical relaxation, and psychological balance.

Massage therapy

A practice where therapists manipulate muscle and connective tissue to enhance function of those tissues and promote relaxation and well-being.

Mind-body medicine

Practices that focus on the interactions among the brain, mind, body, and behavior, with the intent to use the mind to affect physical functioning and promote health.

Mindfulness-based stress reduction (MBSR)

A type of meditation with origins in religious and spiritual traditions. Mindfulness meditation focuses attention on breathing to develop increased awareness of the present. The intent is to reduce stress and control emotions in order to improve health.

Movement-based therapy

The psychotherapeutic use of movement to promote emotional, cognitive, physical, and social integration of individuals.

Musculoskeletal manipulation

Manipulation of the bones and joints, soft tissues, and circulatory and lymphatic systems.

National Center for Complementary and Alternative Medicine (NCCAM)

An agency of the NIH dedicated to exploring complementary and alternative healing practices in the context of rigorous science; training CAM researchers; and disseminating authoritative information to the public and professionals.

National Institutes of Health (NIH)

An agency of the U.S. Department of Health and Human Services that is responsible for biomedical and health-related research.

Olfactory hypnotherapy

A technique that uses scents to arouse potent emotional reactions in the patient. During hypnosis, the patient learns to associate pleasant scents with a sense of security and self-control to overcome phobias and prevent panic attacks.

Pilates

A movement therapy that uses a method of physical exercise to strengthen and build control of muscles, especially those used for posture. Awareness of breathing and precise control of movements are integral components of this approach.

Posttraumatic stress disorder (PTSD)

A severe anxiety disorder that can develop after exposure to any event that results in psychological trauma.

Progressive relaxation

A technique used to relieve tension and stress by systematically tensing and relaxing successive muscle groups.

Prolonged exposure

A form of behavior therapy and cognitive behavioral therapy for PTSD characterized by reexperiencing a traumatic event through remembering it and engaging with reminders of the trauma (triggers).

Qi gong

A practice with origins in Chinese philosophy involving gentle physical movement, mental focus, and deep breathing directed toward specific parts of the body.

Reflexotherapy

A treatment method that uses fingers, needles, and magnet applicators to influence biologically active spots on a human body that are situated where nerve terminals and vessels are concentrated.

Reiki

An energy medicine practice that originated in Japan. In Reiki, the practitioner places hands on or near the person receiving treatment, with the intent to transmit "ki," believed to be life-force energy.

Relaxation therapy

A practice that focuses on using a combination of breathing and muscle relaxation to deal with stress.

Rolfing Structural Integration

A form of deep tissue massage used to realign the tissues that cover and connect all muscles and body organs (fascia). Bringing the body back into proper alignment is thought to reduce pain, improve flexibility and energy, and reduce muscle tension.

Sensory arts therapy

An expressive arts therapy that encourages the patient to express and understand emotions through artistic expression and the creative process.

Serotonin norepinephrine reuptake inhibitors (SNRI)

A class of antidepressant drugs used in the treatment of major depression and other mood disorders. They are sometimes also used to treat anxiety disorders. SNRIs act upon and increase the levels of two neurotransmitters in the brain that are known to play an important part in mood, serotonin and norepinephrine.

Serotonin reuptake inhibitor (SSRI)

A class of medications used to treat psychological conditions including depression and anxiety disorders. SSRIs help increase levels of serotonin in the brain, thus improving mood.

Spinal manipulation

A practice performed by chiropractors and other health care professionals such as physical therapists, osteopaths, and some conventional medical doctors. It involves the use of hands or a device to apply a controlled force to a joint of the spine, moving it beyond its passive range of motion; the amount of force applied depends on the form of manipulation used.

Stress inoculation therapy (SIT)

A cognitive behavioral treatment for PTSD where the goal is to help a patient gain confidence in his or her ability to cope with anxiety and fear stemming from trauma-related reminders. In SIT, the client becomes more aware of reminders for anxiety and fear and learns coping skills that are useful in managing anxiety, such as muscle relaxation and deep breathing.

Tai chi

A mind-body practice, originated in China as a martial art, that involves moving the body in a slow, relaxed, and graceful series of movements. Many practitioners believe that tai chi helps the flow throughout the body of a vital energy called "qi."

Trager Psychophysical Integration

A movement therapy in which practitioners apply a series of gentle, rhythmic rocking movements to the joints. The intent is to release physical tension and increase the body's range of motion.

Trauma-focused therapy

A therapy designed to reduce negative emotional and behavioral responses following child sexual abuse and other traumatic events. The treatment addresses distorted beliefs and attributions related to the abuse and provides a supportive environment in which the patient is encouraged to talk about their traumatic experience.

Whole medical system

A complete system of theory and practice that has evolved over time in different cultures and apart from conventional medicine. Examples of whole medical systems include traditional Chinese medicine, Ayurvedic medicine, homeopathy, and naturopathy.

Yoga

A system of physical postures, breathing techniques, and meditation practiced to promote bodily or mental control and well-being.

www.ingramcontent.com/pod-product-compliance
Lightning Source LLC
Chambersburg PA
CBHW081559170526
45166CB00009B/2751